MW01327372

WARNING

This fresher version of my first book "*Chi Kung Luohan*" makes its content even easier to understand and practice. The original text has now been enlarged and thus, divided into three volumes. This first volume incorporates more information related to the *Taoist* tradition and the seven exercises of the *Tao Yin Han* style, which represent the first section of the *Kung Luohan*, while the second volume presents more detailed information about the *Ba Duan Jin* style or second section of the *Kung Luohan* style and its twelve exercises. This way the reader can concentrate entirely on learning and practicing one section at a time, both complementing the *Kung Luohan Taoist* style. The third volume of this series is about *Tui Na* the therapeutic massage, which is an integral part of a thorough practice of *Kung Luohan*.

On the other hand, I am seeking to provide the reader with more detailed information on each particular topic. Thus, I have removed any information not related to this *Taoist* style, leaving only, those subjects related to the complementing styles.

Since the entire *Kung Luohan* routine is comprised of eighteen exercises plus the *Tui Na*, which have resulted to have certain degree of complexity for the hectic western mind, thus, I have divided it into the three complementing sections. More graphics have been added to this newer version making all the exercises along with their explanation more fluid and easy to comprehend.

The first book was written expecting to provide a clear view of the movements, stances and flow of the routine and to educate the reader about *Chi Kung* in more general terms. If you have the first edition of this book, you do not need to get this newer version, however, if you get it you will find that this presentation has added a more visual explanation.

The reason why I have written this new version, obeys to the fact that many of my students have asked me to make this style's teaching method more accessible and more visually graphic if possible. This is the reason behind this approach.

I hope you find fluid and informative this fresher format and my way of explaining the exercises. Please feel free to visit our Website where you can find photographs and videos of each section.

I also take this opportunity to share with my readers that my book "Cultivating Mindfulness" is an integral part of my teachings. Therefore, the book is absolutely compatible with this and the rest of my works.

In fact, I strongly recommend all my *Chi Kung* students to study said material, which is informative and transformative, and particularly those students who are adopting these teachings to cultivate their nature and character.

Khamrel.

MY APPRECIATION

To my readers for having shared with me their particular interests and needs. This book is the result of such interests and needs.

They asked me to lighten up the first version of *Chi Kung Luohan*, making it more accessible and documented with more graphics.

Those requests have been fulfilled and I look forward to hearing from them about this material, which I strongly believe it will provide students of *Qigong* with clearer textual and graphic explanations.

Keep practicing your *Kung Luohan* routine everyday with enthusiasm and seriousness. Your body and your mind will appreciate your commitment.

Khamrel.

FORWARD

Since I wrote the first version of this topic some years ago many things have happened. In terms of my teaching of this beautiful and somehow challenging art, I have concluded that the people who find these teachings and make them theirs, they change the way they live their everyday lives. *Qigong* is a transformative practice that relates to practitioner's mind-character, body-nature and spirit-consciousness. But only serious, committed and disciplined students, adepts and Cultivators benefit from the treasured gifts *Qigong* has for those who embrace its learning.

Moving into other realms, I have written other books, which have been real challenges since the more one commits to the teaching and learning of this ancient Art, more responsibilities arise and with them our life as adepts and cultivators changes drastically. Cultivating this art is a serious business that cannot be taken for granted. Cultivating our character, our body and our consciousness transcends all we know as ordinary. While ordinary life is what most people know in terms of thinking, feeling, and doing through the waking state of mind.

On the other hand, cultivating is a totally different matter. Cultivation takes you away from ordinariness, centering your consciousness in more subtle realities, which are also here with us, but unseen to the untrained eye. Life then, becomes a real adventure. An adventure that modifies all we know, and which aims toward new horizons. It is an adventure that takes place wherever you are regardless of circumstances in your life. It is very personal, intimate and challenging since it requires your full attention, your unrestricted awareness and committed discipline. How many people you know who are capable of delivering such a commitment to learning?

Throughout my teaching experience I also have come to understand what Master *Ann Liang* told me once..."*Chi Kung* is not for everyone". She meant that many people come and go easily, particularly if they think this is some kind of easy exercise, which promises to improve their health or to give them some supernatural powers. Many people seem to be interested and find ways to learn and practice, although reasons vary, some are somehow superficial, while others are serious.
In my experience I have seen very talented students and some practitioners go astray for not having a clear understanding of this inner urge for learning, and taking all kinds of wicked paths. Also, I have seen students and practitioners developing strong attachments to their practices, transforming their minds in mirrors of affections and dislikes, thus, becoming egotistic and arrogant, unable to distinguish their mental entanglements. However, there are a few students who become true adepts of *Chi Kung*, who seek for assistance and guidance from other students, adepts, and masters, or if they do not find someone around they find the way to rely on their meditation, which always is a superior way.

Have you asked yourself what kind of student are you? What degree of commitment are you willing to put into this learning process? What is burning within your mind and heart, seeking to come out?

Khamrel.

CHAPTER ONE

THE LUOHAN STYLE

Records and tradition tell us that *Siddhartha Gautama Sakyamuni*, the *Buddha*, taught the *Luohan* style originally when he entered into Chinese territories some 500 years before the current era. If this is the case then, the *Luohan* style has a *Buddhist* connotation as well. So, why is it said that this *Qigong* is a *Taoist* style? *Buddhist* and *Taoist* traditions possess similar cultivation methods, both teach that a higher state of consciousness can be achieved through the practice of cultivation (meditation, detachment and care for the body). However, in terms of physical practices the *Buddhist* doctrines teach that the body-mind needs to be cleansed, purified and transformed. For that purpose what does *Taoism* teaches? Guess what? Just the same, therefore, where are the differences? The main differences lay on the type of physical and mental approach to nature's cultivation. That is why there are Traditions!

The *Chi Kung Luohan* style is said to be of *Taoist* origin because it relies on *Qi's* flow through meridians and transmutation of *Qi* through the *Tans* or *Dans*. Also, because it was consistently practiced in *Taoists* monasteries organized and made to meet *Taoist* standards. *Yoga* on the other hand, as practiced in India focuses on performing *Asanas*, which are appropriate to the adept and while performing them he/she meditates. *Qigong* is comprised of stances, movements and breathing techniques that must be rigorously observed. *Qigong's "Li Zhang"* or exercises are soft, gentle and fluid, while *Yoga's asanas* are somehow hard fixed postures practiced along with proper breathing techniques. In both cases, meditation is paramount and its objective is to turn the adept into a mindful and enlightened individual.

The *Kung Luohan* system is comprised of eighteen *Li Zhang*, each one includes stances, movements, breathing and mental focus. Each exercise can be practiced alone, however, it is highly recommended to complete the entire routine, which is divided in two sections. These two sections when practiced separately can be seen as two independent but complementing *Chi Kung* systems by themselves. Thus, they can be practiced separately as two systems or together as one thorough system. I recommend my students to learn each system well and then, put them together as one thorough system. Each of them targets different cultivation aspects; this is why both placed together offer a greater spectrum of benefits.

For those who are at the beginning of their learning, the first section of this whole system is called *Tao Yin Han* and it is comprised of seven exercises. The most relevant aspect of it is the use of sound frequencies and vibration or resonance in the form of specific syllables, expressed while exhaling. This is why this style is also known as "the Six Healing Sounds *Qigong*".

These six different sounds are simple and should not be related or compared to "*mantras*". The sounds used in this *Qigong* style are specific personal vibratory frequencies that target the three large bodily cavities or burners in which organs and glands are found.

Sound vibration or resonance acts as an internal massage which, when reaching the organs and glands make them respond to it, either helping them to heal if sick, or reestablishing their functions if these have been diminished, or even invigorating their performance if they are healthy. These are the properties of the healing frequencies!

For practical reasons, these sounds whether they are practiced alone or along with the *Li Zhang* or exercises, they must be clear, loud and clean. This means that the student and adept must inhale slowly and deeply releasing his exhalation thoroughly by producing the sound, this way, a clear and almost tangible vibration is to be felt somewhere within the body. This resonance will have a positive effect upon organs and glands reached by the sound's vibration-frequency.

Another very important aspect of the practice is the breathing technique. Serious practitioners of *Yoga* and *Qigong* all over the ages have understood this relevant matter. Deep breathing, natural breathing, diaphragmatic breathing or *Buddha*'s breathe and reverse breath are techniques that require the practitioner to use his/her diaphragm fully while inhaling and exhaling. Which means that in the process of breathing, the lungs are filled fully and emptied totally, invigorating and working out the Psoas muscle.

However, this process needs to be done slowly so the breath can be followed, measured and experienced consciously. It must be observed that the deeper and slower the breath, the better performed the exercises will be. In this regard we have two axioms to remember; "Energy follows Thought" and "Movement follows Breath".

When practicing this first section of the *Kung Luohan* system, the lungs are filled fully allowing the student/adept to exhale and produce the sounds in a large capacity, experiencing the vibration internally and being able to locate the body cavity where organs and glands are located. In regards to this matter, there are three main areas or bodily cavities where organs are located, underneath the

diaphragm (abdomen), above the diaphragm (chest) and the neck-head.
The second section or *Ba Duan Jin,* which will be presented in Volume II of this series, is comprised of twelve exercises and the most relevant aspect of it is the use of bodily vibration produced by the limbs while performing specific movements in each exercise. This means that each exercise or *Li Zhang* posses this vibratory element in it and must be done without any reservation. This bodily vibration acts upon the nervous system, more specifically upon the "Vagus" nerve, which is the core of the autonomic nervous system, connecting with all organs and glands, nurturing and making them to function. Also the deep breathing technique will allow the practitioner to perceive the flow of energy moving through the meridians and orbits.
As to the third section or *Tui Na*, which is to be presented in Volume III of this series, follows a bodily diagram that allows the awakened *Qi* to move through the meridian system, removing energy clogs, widening obstructed meridians and invigorating acupuncture points. This system of therapeutic massage employs the same principles used in acupuncture with the difference that we use our hands to apply pressure upon the meridians and pressure points.
Now, it is important to mention that sound-frequency, bodily vibration, acupressure and breath are fundamental for obtaining the physical and mental benefits that the *Kung Luohan* system promises to its adepts. And why is this possible? Well, something the old Chinese and other ancient cultures knew about the body is nowadays being rediscovered through medical science. These ancient cultures knew so much about these matters that they not only devised ways for approaching and healing their

bodies when appropriate, but they also discovered their intimate interactions with nature and how their bodies reacted because of the different aspects of cause and effect. To those cultures life was simple and very close to nature, thus, maintaining their bodies fit was easier. Also, their views of life were different, they had a different understanding of how life evolved and how intimately related to the planet it was.

Although, this ancient understanding was different to our current way of perceiving and handling our lives, the fundamental principles are still the same. Despite the fact that our lives are more complicated and our relationship to the planet and all its intricacies are far distant, still, we are living beings product of what this the planet is made of. We are human beings consisting of physical, mental, emotional and energy aspects or bodies, the same as the ancient human beings. Perhaps the reasons why we have developed weird and devastating diseases are because we have walked away from our natural source and awakened consciousness. We treat nature as something that belong to us, destroying it in the name of economics, altering it because we can through technological development, polluting and using it as we please and this is a very wrong approach, thus, we are reducing ourselves to extinction.

FLOW OF QI

In previous paragraphs I have mentioned that *Qi* flows through a system of meridians or energy channels. This system is made of energy, however, its energy paths follow the nervous ramifications as well as the veins and arteries that crisscross the entire body. It can be said that this energy system reaches every single cell within the body. This is how the entire human body is nurtured with energy or *Qi*. We must remember that *Qi* is the life force that

keeps our bodily systems functioning and our consciousness awake, and that we are not the source of *Qi* but just a medium through which, *Qi* flows to evolve.
According to the Traditional Chinese medicine (TCM) there are three main channels that permit the flow of *Qi* to reach all organs and cells and they are:

(A) The *Zhong Mai* channel, which runs through the center of the human body, bisecting it along a vertical axis and goes along with the Vagus nerve. It can be pictured as connecting the center of the skull (*Bahui* acupoint) to the perineum (*Hui Yin* acupoint).

(B) The *Ren Mai* channel, which runs along the front part of the human body. It is responsible for channeling the *Yin* polarity. It passes through the tongue and apex of the sternum, and

(C) The *Du Mai* channel, which runs along the back part of the human body. It follows the Spinal Cord, and it is responsible for channeling the *Yang* polarity.

These three energy circuits have their confluence points at the top of the head, the crown or *Bahui* acupoint and the perineum or *Hui Yin* acupoint. Furthermore, these three channels are interconnected, and give way to small, large and borderline orbits, which move *Qi* through the body by following specific energy paths.
Deriving from these three channels are twelve energy pathways, also known as meridians and countless smaller tributaries, which manifest energetically within the entire human body. Each of these twelve conduits in turn correspond to one of the twelve vital organs, thus, these energy channels or meridians travel through the body reaching each vital organ-gland. The tributaries reach the rest of body cells.

However, there is another very important energy channel or should I say, “belt”. It moves horizontally as the parallels of planet Earth, and they also assist the human body with *Qi* and divide the body in quadrants.
Practicing *Qigong* helps to maintain health, flexibility, strength and functionality of these meridians, distributing vital energy to the physical and mental bodies. Ultimately, being healthy consists in having the meridians completely harmonic and with normal *Qi* flow. Any saturation, blockage or damage of these channels can cause disease, sickness or even death.
Since the moment we are in our mother’s womb, we are receiving *Qi* through the maternal fountain and once we take our first breathe then; we begin absorbing *Qi* by our own capacity. At this moment the *Qi* is bipolar, meaning that it has two charges *Yang* and *Yin* coexisting in equal amounts or in equilibrium, clean, clear and balanced. Our capacity to breathe becomes natural and *Qi* begins to move through our body as oxygen flows through our lungs and arteries reaching every single cell. The human body possess its own ways of storing *Qi*, however, this *Qi* may become corrupted and needs to be exchanged frequently with fresh *Qi*.
Our *Qi* flows through the meridians as said before, reaching every organ and gland nurturing them entirely. As we age we develop and acquire all sorts of emotional, mental and physical vices, corrupted mental notions and thousands of attachments of all kinds. This corruption of mind and body also affects the quality of our *Qi*. This corrupted flow of *Qi* quickly loses its *Yang* charge and the space before occupied by the *Yang* polarity is replaced by the *Yin* polarity, thus, our energy balance is compromised and in some cases, lost and more health problems emerge along with age, getting fragile and in poor health.

Due to this depletion of *Yang* energy-polarity, mature, intelligent, and prudent people must assume great responsibility towards cultivating their remaining *Yang* energy. This is why we learn *Qigong*; by practicing it one can care for, recuperate, accumulate, store, expand and balance his/her *Yang* polarity; thus, recuperating our health, strength, vitality and promoting physical, emotional and mental fitness, reducing or eliminating diseases and slowing down the aging process (longevity).

If an individual can learn and practice *Qigong*, he will be able to generate, store and use *Yang* energy from what little still remains in his reservoir well beyond the age of sixty. Not only will health be recuperated, but also internal organs, glands and bodily systems will also rejuvenate, and in general, all cells will benefit greatly. In other words, any person can practice *Qigong* no matter age or physical condition; even convalescent people can practice it.

The practice of *Qigong* may take place at any moment of the day and the physical place where it is practiced may be small or large, lighted or dark, the only thing that is recommended is to have good ventilation. The practice of *Qigong* makes emphasis in a lifestyle of measured behavior according to age. Harmonizing your way of life with your age not only maintains good health, it helps to heal many dysfunctions that an aging body might develop.

Previously, I mentioned that the meridian system also has energy centers; these *Tans* or *Chakras* transmute the flow of energy into higher frequencies. These vortexes, energy centers, *chakras* or *tans* vary according to traditions. Some say that the human body possesses countless number of energy vortexes, others point to nine, seven or even three. In our tradition we concentrate on three main *Tans* or *Dans,* and some other energy vortexes that are reached while performing the exercises of the system.

It is relevant to know *Tans'* location since it helps us to focus our attention through the practice and these are:

(A) *Tan Tien* or lower *Dantien*, located in the area known as the navel or lower abdomen, in between the belly button, the perineum and the sacrum-coccyx.

(B) *Tan Zhong* or middle *Dantien*, located right at the bottom or lower tip of the sternum, just behind the bone and underneath the diaphragm, sometimes known as the heart *chakra*, and

(C) *Tan Mu* or higher *Dantien*, located in between the eyebrows and in the middle of the brain, also known as the pineal *chakra.*

Hereby, we can notice that each of these *Tans* is present in each of the body's large cavities or burners before mentioned.

Now, about these other energy vortexes I just mentioned. They are located usually in pairs (*Yin-Yang*) and are easily found. However, it is not necessary to think about them since they open their flow once we begin consciously practicing the movements. These points are usually considered acupuncture points and their relevance is well known. In our practice, we do not touch these points, however, our hands constantly glide over them and this slight-energy-touch is enough for activating them.

The function of these vortexes is precisely to attract and emit energy. They absorb *Qi* from the environment integrating it into the meridian system and once the *Qi* flows through the body and *Tans* where it gets transmuted into higher frequencies, then is transported and stored in all cells, while some may be expelled through these vortexes. Humans also absorb and exchange *Qi* through their breath.

KUNG LUOHAN KEY ASPECTS

When performing any of the three sections pertaining to the *Kung Luohan* style, the student and practitioner must observe certain key aspects that are relevant to the results experienced from practicing a true *Qigong* tradition. These principles are:

1. All movements, no matter how minute they are, must carry your full attention: Careful and coordinated movements are elements of a fluid and balanced performance.

2. Rhythmic breathing: "Movement follows breath", which must be deep, slow and coordinated with all movements. Inhaling means stretching and exhaling means contracting. However, while practicing the *Tao Yin Han* or first section, exhalation produces the sound no matter if we are stretching some body parts.

3. Awakened state of mind: Being fully aware of stance, sounds, movements and breath produces a meditative state of mind.

4. Movements and stances, although miniscule are fundamentally important: Head-Eyes-Tongue, arms-hands, legs-feet and torso play an absolute important role. Nothing can be left unattended.

5. Mental alertness quiets the mind: An idling mind must be prevented at all times by remaining aware of yourself and the environment. It helps to visualize mental or external object(s), sensing *Qi*'s flow, introspection of philosophical concepts, and connection to natural objects, and creative positive imagination.

6. Softness and gentleness: Relaxed muscles and soft facial expression, fluid movements through permanent observation.

7. Solid posture: Straight vertebral column through tilting-in both chin and pelvis, well rooted stance.

8. Seeking for oscillating balance and counterbalance: All movements sprang from body's center of gravity, observing symmetric equilibrium in all movements.

9. Students and practitioners must observe throughout all their practices the following states:

- Equanimity through fluid and relaxed movements;
- Tranquility through calm and relaxed mind;
- Calmness through nearly imperceptible movements, "the slower the better".

CRESTS & VALLEYS

Another fundamental aspect of our practice that needs to be understood is the permanent equilibrium of contrary or opposing forces or movements at play. Examples of this condition are the progressive extension and contraction of limbs and joints, or the tensing and relaxing of muscles, or the inhalation and exhalation of air, all always done to a complete extent. This alternation between the two polarities *Yin* and *Yang* is what we have referred as to "Crests and Valleys" and in a more practical way, "Oscillation", which also shows the intermittent flow of cycles in all levels of life.

The sought balance also shows a cycle that looks to soften the flow of *Qi* and other bodily fluids throughout the body, making the student and adept more conscious of their own relaxation and tension in a more tangible way. In this

manner, each person can control the flow of bodily fluids until mental stillness is achieved. Simply put, each movement has its counterpart. The duality reflects the *Yin-Yang* principle as one element is incorporated into the other. If it goes up, it then comes down; if it stretches, it then contracts; if it grows, it then shrinks; if it tenses, it then relaxes, and so on.
When practicing any of the three sections, or all three consecutively, the student and adept must observe the following cycles:

* Inhale when stretching the limbs and exhale when contracting them.
* Inhale when moving to the left and exhale when moving to the right.
* Inhale when stretching backwards and exhale when bending forward.
* Inhale when stretching up and exhale when shrinking.
* Inhale when stretching back and exhale when bending over.
* Inhale while attracting *Qi* and exhale when applying pressure upon a body part.
* Inhale while relaxing and exhale when rubbing or shaking.

To avoid the accumulation of tension and bodily fluids, exhalation must not last longer than inhalation. The breath cycle should be even and always closely connected to the movements; remember, "movement follows breath". Beginners will find helpful to keep control over their breath cycle and movements by 'counting'. You may adopt the custom of counting from one to nine as the basis for practicing each movement. This measure is based on what is known as the *Yang* cycle. Everything that exists within the *Yang* cycle originates as one and ends at nine, it then journeys back until it arrives at one again, and begins a new count, persisting as an endless cycle. In this manner, *Yang* energy gradually fills the body with *Qi* charged with *Yang* polarity, which generally speaking, older people lack.

The *Kung Luohan* style is also known in China as "the enlightened art of breathing". Practiced regularly, it helps activate the intrinsic flow of vital energy through the meridians, it strengthens organs and glands, it gives vitality to body and mind, it exercises muscles, and it promotes relaxation and manages stress. This particular style also enhances attentiveness. *Kung Luohan* promotes the harmonization and merging of *Yin* and *Yang* polarities to "dispel wicked forces" from the body, and to allow the "original *Qi*" to be purified.

The self-healing effects of a continuous practice will make the body healthy. A transcendental purpose for practicing *Kung Luohan* is to recuperate and balance the lacking *Yang* polarity.

THE SIX HEALING SOUNDS

A primary application of the Six Healing Sounds is to aid in correcting any emotional disharmony caused by the stress of modern life. The Six Healing Sounds also called *Liuzijue*, is a breathing technique devised by the ancient Chinese to improve health and promote healing and longevity. The earliest record of this breathing technique is believed to have been developed by *Tao Hongjing*, a well known Traditional Chinese Medicine doctor, Taoist, alchemist as well as astrologer who lived from 456 to 536 c.e.

According to the Traditional Chinese Medicine (TCM), the five major organs or *Zhang* organs — heart, liver, spleen, lung and kidney — are each assigned a natural element which are: Wood, Fire, Earth, Metal, Water, which were the names chosen to describe the five types of "elemental energies". Trees (wood) come to life in the spring. Fire is hot like the summer. Earth is most fertile in late summer/early autumn. In winter there is much rain and snow and water freezes.

Basic correspondences were found between these elemental energies and the five organ systems of the human body. Liver and Wood are both flexible and smooth. The Heart like a Fire warms the entire body. Earth grows food, which the Spleen-stomach digests. Metal is cool and hard and is used to make containers, thus, the Lungs are also cool and encased in a hard rib cage, containing the breath (sick lungs also resemble badly rusted iron).

Every organ also has an associated sound with which the organ resonates. By using the associated sound, stale and congested *Qi* can be expelled from the affected organ and be replaced with fresh, clear and healthy *Qi*. When *Qi* gets rancid and/or blocked due to inappropriate diet, poor lifestyle habits, repressed emotions and/or weak constitution, it becomes congested and turns into a cause of pain, discomfort or illness.

Depending on where the *Qi* gets stuck symptoms vary. If it gets stuck in the spleen the stale *Qi* may manifest as bloating, abdominal pain, gas, and/or poor digestion. If it is stuck in the liver then, it might be felt as pain in the lower right rib cage, manifesting as quick temper or liver/gallbladder dysfunction. If it gets trapped in the head then, it could lead to headache or illusion. According to TCM theories, badly congested *Qi* can also lead to stagnated blood and blood clots.

Practicing the Six Healing Sounds help to move out congested *Qi* and allow the body to get rid of it by creating different internal vibrations and pressures within different large cavities and organs. In other words, when you pronounce the six healing sounds you are giving the internal organs a good massage and expelling the stale *Qi*.

There are a few ways for using the six healing sounds, and its usage largely depends on your current state of health:

(1) For health maintenance: Practice the six healing sounds in this order, which is based on the mutual generation of the five elements: Xū (Wood) → Hēng (Fire) → Hū (Earth) → Ha (Metal) → Shuī (Water) → Xī (Wood).

(2) To promote healing: Practice the six healing sounds in the order based on the mutual overcoming of the five elements: Heng (Fire) → Ha (Metal) → Xū (Wood) → Hū (Earth) → Shuī (Water) → Xī (Wood).

(3) To promote physical and mental alignment or centeredness: Practice the six healing sounds in the following order: {Heng (Fire) → Hu (Earth)} → {Heng (Fire) → Ha (Metal)} → Shui (Water) → Ha (Metal) → Xi (Wood) → {Heng (Fire) → Ha (Metal)} → {Xu (Wood) → Hu (Earth)}.

Alternatively, if you are short of time for a full practice you can practice just the sound that is associated with the current season. For example, if it is winter, practice the sound "Shuī" to strengthen the kidney system. Note that the last sound Xī can be practiced all year round to support the triple burner.

Regardless of whether you are practicing all six healing sounds or only one of them, always breathe in slowly through your nose and breathe out evenly through the pronouncing of the sound through your mouth. Repeat each sound three, six or nine times, and practice the sequence (be it one sound or six sounds) preferably three times a day.

The early version of the Six Healing Sounds was merely a breathing technique that did not include any movements. But as it evolved through time, movements were added to aid in the flow of *Qi* and to better expel stale *Qi* out of the body. Each set of assisting moves (*Tao Yin Han*) is gentle and easy to learn for young and old alike.

As we know, *Tao Yin Han* is a series of movements where each one of them has a corresponding sound. Throughout all *Tao Yin Han* movements keep yourself calm and composed and your movements fluid, controlled and coordinated with your breathing and the healing sounds.

The general guideline says: Beginners should pronounce each healing sound out loud. That means audible sound should be produced when you are practicing each syllable. This will help you to get the right pronunciation, prevent the holding of breath and familiarize you with flow of *Qi* that each sound makes within the body. As you become more familiar with the different vibrations produced by each sound, whether or not an audible sound is made becomes less important. The importance, after all, is not the sound itself, but how it is produced. At this stage, if you find that little or no sound is made during your practice it is perfectly all right. Inhale through the nose and loudly or silently make the sounds as you exhale through the mouth.

The seven sets of *Tao Yin Han* movements are preceded by opening or preliminary moves called *Qi Shi* to activate the *Qi*, and end with finishing moves called *Shou Shi* to guide *Qi* back to the lower *Tan Tian*; the navel area where life-force is gathered and stored.

One important aspect of mingling the sounds and movements is that the energy or *Qi* gets activated initially

through the *Qi Shi* then, moved through the meridians and orbits by the exercises or movements of the *Tao Yin Han*, and through the sounds, their frequencies and vibrations reach the targeted organs and glands. This is a compound workout, energy distribution, synchronized movement; frequencies, vibration and resonance are combined to produce wellbeing, to amplify consciousness and to improve health.
These are the six healing sounds, practice them as a group or separately, while sitting or while practicing the *Li Zhang* of the *Tao Yin Han*:

Xu (Shuu) sound, is associated to the liver organ, the wood element and spring season. When exhaling do it loudly producing the sound, and by using the breath-mind-imagination lead and guide the *Qi* from the inner sides of the big toes up the insides of the thighs, into the abdomen, up to the throat, eyes, forehead, to the crown of the head; then back down into the lungs, then down the inner sides of the arms, ending in the outer tips of the thumbs.
Then inhale and repeat 3, 6 or 9 times. The Liver helps to control the quality of the blood, and supports the eyesight.

He (Heng) sound is associated to the heart organ, the fire element and summer season. When exhaling do it loudly producing the sound, and by using the breath-mind-imagination, lead and guide the *Qi* from the outer sides of the big toes, up the inner legs into the abdomen to the upper chest, armpits, and along the inner arms to the inside tips of the little fingers.
Then inhale and repeat 3, 6 or 9 times. The Heart controls the circulation of blood. The *Tan Zhong* or Heart energy center is the location of fire, which if in excess can bring about the stagnation or deficiency of the blood, as well as profoundly affecting how well the mind is working. Some

suggest that the use of sound will assist in the healing of heart diseases as well as mental disturbances.

Hu (Huu) sound, is associated to the spleen organ, the earth element and all seasons. When exhaling do it loudly producing the sound, guiding the *Qi* upward from the outer sides of the big toes, up the inner-legs into the abdomen to the stomach, then into upper chest where it divides into two flows: (1) Brings the *Qi* to the throat and under the tongue. Simultaneously, (2) moves the *Qi* into the inner arms down to the inside tips of the little fingers.
Then inhale and repeat 3, 6 or 9 times. Stomach digests food. Spleen helps transporting the nutrients and the related *Qi*-energy of food.

Ha (Haa or Tzz) sound, is associated to the lungs organ, the metal element and autumn season. When exhaling do it loudly producing the sound, guiding the *Qi* upward from the inner sides of the big toes, up the inner legs, into the abdomen, into the lungs; then down the inner arms to the inner portions of the tips of both thumbs (Lung-11 acupressure point).
Then inhale and repeat 3, 6, or 9 times. Lungs of all the five organ-systems are the organs with more contact with the outer world and with all its negative pathogenic influences, such as germs, viruses, and illness causing pollutants. Also the lungs bring in the rich *Qi* of the air, which is so absolutely vital for life itself.

Chui (Shui or chwai) sound, is associated to the kidneys organ, the water element and winter season. When exhaling do it loudly producing the sound, guiding the *Qi* upward from the balls of the feet or *Yong Chuan* (Kidney-1 point), through the inner thighs, along the spine, into the kidneys, into the chest, down the inner arms into the tips of the middle fingers (Pericardium-9).

Then inhale and repeat 3, 6, or 9 times. The Kidneys oversee many functions needed for wellbeing. Some of the most important are reproduction, urination, general vitality, and psychological factors such as memory.

Xi (Shii) sound is associated to the triple burner - digestive and gallbladder organs, the wood element, and all seasons. When exhaling do it loudly producing the sound, guiding the *Qi* upward from the outer tips of the fourth toes (Gall Bladder-44) along the outer legs, into the sides of the torso, to the sides of the neck and into the head; then down the sides of the head, neck, shoulders, and back of the arms to the outside tips of the ring fingers (Triple Burner-1). Then, continue on with the inhalation by "Going in reverse". Move the *Qi* back from the tips of the ring fingers, up the back of the arms, to the shoulders, then neck, to the head, down the sides of head, neck, sides of torso into the outer legs to finish where you started at the ends of the fourth toes (GB-44). Repeat up to nine times.

Note: The triple burner, warmer or energizer, also called *San Jiao*, refers not to a physical organ but to the energetic pathways that run through the upper (neck-head), middle (chest) and lower (abdomen) large cavities of the body. One of its main functions is to regulate *Qi* and fluids surrounding the internal organs. The Triple Burner refers to the functioning not the physicality of the organs of the body. The sound used for the Triple Burner aids in harmonizing all of these functions. The Upper Burner has the lungs, heart and the brain. The Middle Burner has the spleen, pancreas stomach and the liver. Here food is metabolized for energy and cell growth. The Lower Burner refers to the area of the kidneys, bladder, and intestines, areas that deal with the elimination of waste.

Traditional Chinese Medicine believes that mental and physical problems are caused by *Qi*-energy imbalances in the organs and meridians. Since the Six Sounds are said to rectify such imbalances, it is easy to see why this *Qigong* practice has become so popular in several societies.

THE RELEVANCE OF DEEP BREATHE

We call our way of breathing in many ways, some of them are: natural breathing, diaphragmatic breathing, abdominal breathing, belly breathing, *Buddha* breath or baby breathing. When we breathe 'deeply', the incoming air that passes through our nose fully fills our lungs, starting at the bottom thus; we will notice that our lower belly rises. Then, the inhaled air keeps filling up the lungs until they are fully filled, lightly expanding the thorax.

The ability to breathe so deeply and powerfully is an ability nourished by those who meditate. This skill is available to everyone and comes along with newborns but more than often lies dormant. Reawakening it allows you to activate several of your body's strongest self-healing mechanisms.

So, why does practicing deep breathing seem so unnatural to many of us? One reason that can be found at the beginning of our lives lies on our prejudicial culture, which more than often encourages us for hiding our emotions, which are linked to our thinking. This kind of emotional restriction or limitation alters brain waves that unconsciously make us to hold our breath or breath irregularly. Other factual alterations are fashion and body image. People tend to think that a sculptured body should not show a prominent stomach, thus, restricting deep breath and making shallow "chest breathing" becomes, looks and feels normal. This kind of holding our breath generates tension and anxiety due to the fact that our brain receives less oxygen.

The act of breathing draws the diaphragm, a powerful layer of muscle that divides the chest cavity from the abdominal cavity. As you breathe in, the diaphragm pushes downward, pulling the lungs with it and pressing against the Psoas muscle and abdominal organs to make room for the expanded lungs as they fill with air. As you breathe out, the diaphragm presses back upward against the lungs, helping to expel carbon dioxide. Shallow breathing limits the diaphragm's range of motion to a very small portion, which is the upper portion of the lungs and never gets a full share of oxygenated air, preventing cells from receiving enough oxygen. That can make you feel tired, short of breath, nervous and anxious. However, deep breathing sends the incoming air to the lowest portion of the lungs, which is where many small blood vessels reside, and air keeps filling up the lungs with more air.
Deep abdominal breathing encourages full oxygen exchange, which means that the beneficial trade of incoming oxygen for outgoing carbon dioxide takes place. This type of deep breathing slows the heartbeat and can lower or stabilize blood pressure.

Here is how to take a deep, healing, diaphragmatic breath:

First step: Place yourself in a comfortable and quiet place then stand still, sit or lie down. Start by observing the length of your breath. First take a normal breath then, try taking a slower, deeper breath. The air coming in through your nose should move downward into the lower section of your lungs. Let your abdomen expand fully. Now breathe out through your nose, which is the natural way.
Alternate normal and deep breaths several times. Pay attention to how you feel when you inhale and exhale normally and when you breathe deeply. Shallow breathing often feels tense and constricted and can be noticed by the expansion of the chest, while deep breathing produces

relaxation and can be noticed by the slight expansion of the belly. Increase your practice for several minutes.

Second step: Place one hand on your abdomen, just below your belly button. Feel your hand rise about an inch each time you inhale and fall about an inch each time you exhale. Your chest will barely expand, in concert with your abdomen. Remember to relax your belly so that each inhalation expands it fully.

Third step: Once you have taken the first two steps, you can move on to regular practice of focusing your mind. As you sit on *Zazen* or Lotus or stand on *Wu Ji* or *Daikou* comfortably with your eyes open or closed, blend your breathing with:

(1) While breathing: employ an image, a word or a phrase that helps you relax and focus your attention on. Then, visualize that the air you breathe in washes peace and quiet into your body and as you breathe out, imagine that the air leaving your body carries tension and anxiety away with it. As you inhale, repeat this phrase to yourself: "Breathing in brings peace and quiet." And as you exhale, say: "Breathing out takes away tension and anxiety."

NOTE: It is reasonable to start with 3 minutes of breath focus and gradually add time. However, once you engage in practicing your *Tao Yin Han* routine the deep breathing will be part of it. Once you become used to this kind of breathing its regular practice will become natural to you.

(2) Moving breathing: begin moving by following the *Li Zhang* or exercises of your routine. Start with the preliminary movements. Every time you expand or stretch you breathe in and every time you contract or bend you breathe out, or simply follow the directions of the exercise. Your mind follows this continuous flow without judging whatever you are doing; remove thoughts from your mind by observing the flow of breath and movement.

A wide variety of benefits are experienced when we include deep breathing to our daily exercises and to our regular lifestyle. This extraordinary practice should be done throughout the day or whenever you find yourself with stress, upset, pain or feeling tired. The more you practice the deep breathing, the more natural you will feel it, thus, improving your mental and bodily functions.

Everyday our body gets exposed to many harmful substances, toxins and other things that may provoke cell and tissue damage, this is why during deep breath exhalation stage, the body will exhale the toxins which are bound by the hemoglobin inside the red blood cells, cleaning up the blood. And during the inhalation stage the body absorbs more oxygen, which is the main component in the metabolism process within the cells, this way it helps in repairing the cells and tissue.

When our body gets more oxygen, it increases metabolism rate and gives us more energy as well as calming our brain from craving food by controlling the production of weight regulating hormone, leptin and ghrelin. Deep breathing brings in more oxygen into the body, which is needed by all bodily functions and cells. The incoming oxygen helps to remove the neurotransmitter within the blood that induces pain caused by nerve or blood circulatory conditions.

Also, the incoming oxygen helps the body to relieve anxiety by promoting the production of endorphins. Whereas, endorphins are hormones which promote feeling happiness and comfort, they can make us feel good, fresh and happy even after a stressful day, thus, it is recommended to practice deep breathing when you feel tense or stressed.

Deep breathing also increases the blood ability to shield the oxygen and prevent it from binding the carbon monoxide, which is a toxin, found in the air and in exhalation. During exhalation, the air expelled is full of toxins contained and gathered from the blood. Deep breathing helps in cleaning the blood from any harmful substance and metabolic waste such as carbon dioxide and carbon monoxide. The more oxygen we get, the stronger the body immune system gets.
Deep breathing exercise promotes the production of more healing substances such as hormones, proteins, enzymes, etc., and improves the immune cells function in fighting diseases. The deep breathing exercises also help to improve the lungs capacity and functions. Practicing deep breathing exercises regularly improve and maintain normal functioning of the nervous system. By bringing more oxygen to the brain it helps to calm the brain nerves, which lead to migraine pain reduction.
Deep breathing method also helps to calm the nerves and induces the production of melatonin, the hormone that makes you sleepy. Also, during deep breathing practice, the lungs, diaphragm, Psoas muscle, heart, liver and other organs get massaged, helping them to improve their functioning. Remember that lungs are one of the main excretory organs in the body. They play an important role in flushing away toxins that are present in blood.
Deep breathing will not only promote better oxygenation but, it also induce the body to exhale more stale air which contains many waste and toxins substances derived from the inner body realm. Practicing deep breathing techniques will help to clear the mind and facilitate focusing at whatever we do. Practicing deep breathing exercises while sitting or standing and holding the back straight can help to improve body posture as well as prevent from scoliosis.

In summary, deep breathing practice offers many great effects including the following: It treats symptoms of menopause and treats cancer side effects; it reduces pain, relieves anxiety and alleviates stress; it helps in quitting smoking and drinking; it cleans the blood and strengthens muscles and immune system; it improves posture, blood quality and lungs function; it promotes good mood and repairs cell damage; it helps in weight control; it increases nerve functions and relieves migraine; it induces good sleep and maintains organs health; it gets rid of toxins and clears the mind among other less obvious benefits.

These are just a few physical beneficial effects; still there is plenty mental positive effect that will be discussed later.

Practicing deep breathing exercises have no actual side effects other than hyperventilation, which will make you feel dizzy for a few seconds, however, as soon as you feel it, just slow down or limit your breathe intake for a few seconds, or lower your head below the heart level and you will be fine again. Fast or accelerated breathing or too deep breathing is the cause of hyperventilation. Deep breathing exercises can also make you experience sleepiness, light-headache, hand and face tingling sense, and altered consciousness. If you get any of these side effects sensations just relax and slow your breath.

Whenever you decide to practice the deep breathing exercise start by doing it slowly to avoid the negative side effects. By practicing deep breathing slowly, you will enjoy the benefits of it and later you may increase the time, speed and intensity of your deep breathing. Whenever you feel ready for longer practice periods, you can extend the depth. Watch the side effects and stop when you feel any awkward sensation.

Lastly, but not less important is what I have to say about how to manage your own deep breath when practicing the

Qi exercises or *Li Zhang*. A few paragraphs before I mentioned that most people have forgotten how to properly breathe, and because of such a mischievous neglect, people suffer from all sorts of maladies. However, when people decide to practice *Qigong*, one of their first learning tasks is to remember how to breathe and thus, they begin practicing the above mentioned breathing exercises. Sooner than later, people find that their lungs capacity is not enough for accomplishing all the exercises as prescribed, particularly speaking, about the deep breath sequences.

People find that when inhaling, their movements do not reach the required stretch and when exhaling their contraction is not enough and then, they got frustrated and quit their practice and perhaps they end their interest for *Qigong*. Then, what to do when a situation like this arises?

First, you have to be calm and patient with your body and mind, constantly observing the synchronicity of your movements with the length of your deep breath cycle. And secondly, you should try lowering the speed of your breath cycle (inhalation-exhalation) and see if it helps to complete the movements along the deep breath cycle. Remember that lungs are flexible sacks of muscle and they need to regain their natural flexibility again.

If it does not change then, try splitting the movements so you can catch up with your breath. Fortunately, most exercises allow this kind of break, allowing the student to merge the movement with the breath cycle without altering the flow of energy.

CHAPTER TWO

GETTING READY FOR PRACTICE

Many students and some practitioners become concerned with lots of unimportant elements and most of the time these worries are the product of misinformation, old rigid mental notions or emotional attachments, sometimes called superstition. True adepts must eventually get rid of all kinds of mental, emotional and physical attachments and particularly, superstitious attachments. Therefore, there are no limitations or impositions concerning our daily practice. Just a few simple recommendations:

Practice cycle: You may practice any of the three sections of the *Kung Luohan* style, consecutively or separately at any moment of the day; however, practicing during the early morning hours or at sunset or afterwards enhances your discipline and wellbeing. If the whole routine takes longer than expected you can always divide it in shorter segments.
When you had fully learned the first section (*Tao Yin Han*) you must practice it regularly (daily if possible) and thoroughly until you had learned the second and third sections. Once all sections had been learned they must be practiced together if possible, however, each section can be practiced separately but all should be practiced daily. You can even divide each section if practice time is of concern.

Practice comfort: It is suggested to wear light, flexible and breathable clothes and footwear. Avoid eating just before your practice and wait at least twenty minutes after finishing your practice for your next meal. Do not drink cold water either before or right after your practice, wait at least twenty minutes to drink water at room temperature.

Also, do not shower right after your practice, again, wait at least 20 minutes. Always retain a nice smile and a positive attitude. The reason behind these preventions is that, if resting time is not allowed after each practice the generated, distributed and accumulated *Qi* will be disrupted and wasted.

Practice facilities: It is not necessary to practice in a *Dojo, Ashram* or *Zendo*. Any place is perfect for practicing your *Kung Luohan* routine. As a matter of fact, a small site is good enough. Take into consideration that in ancient times hermit monks used to practice their routine in very small cottages. You can practice in a room, garden, park or any other well-ventilated place. Illumination, particular flooring or electricity are of no importance. I do not recommend the use of incense, music or other elements, which may distract you or even worse, these elements may create an attachment difficult to eradicate in the future. However, it is suggested to find a pleasant well-ventilated place; tranquility and minimum distractions are a plus.

Practice rhythm: I have mentioned before “movement follows breathe” and, that “the slower the movement, the better”. This means that if you are aware of your breath’s length you can adjust your movements’ speed, and wherever your attention goes your internal energy follows.

Practice length: It is recommended by *Sifus* and Masters to observe the required repetitions, which usually are recommended within each exercise explanation. When the beginner student follows this rule, the complete *Tao Yin Han* section, which is comprised, of 7 exercises can be completed in between 5 and 10 minutes. While the *Ba Duan Jin* section*, which has 12 exercises,* can be done in between 20 and 50 minutes. Tui Na may be completed in between 5 and 10 minutes. In all cases you can always extend the number of repetitions of each exercise by adding multiples of nine repetitions.

Once you know all 18 movements of the *Kung Luohan* routine, plus the therapeutic *Tui Na* massage then, you could complete it in between 40 minutes to an hour and a half depending on your breathe capacity and movements fluidity. However, seasoned practitioners may adjust their routines depending on their awareness, energy sensitivity, time availability and other factors that may alter a full routine schedule.

It is also recommended not exceeding 90 minutes of practice a day. Anytime between 30 to 90 minutes is a reasonable practice time. It is fundamentally important to practice everyday. Literature regarding *Chi Kung* usually mentions the idea that “the conscious, alert and discerning mind is the greatest player in this matter”, and that “cultivating the *Tan Tien* (elixir) requires hard work during a period of time before it can be harvested”. Grand Master *Che T'Ong* had mentioned that 90 continuous days of serious hard work, would reveal the treasures of *Wai Tan Kung Luohan*. To establish the fundamentals, at least 90 days of disciplined practice are required.

This means that only after 90 days of daily and committed practice the student and practitioner will experience and see tangible results.

PRACTICE RECOMMENDATIONS

Concentration: Whenever the student or practitioner engages in his/her daily practice mental focus, attentiveness and sight are crucial to the postures. To facilitate concentration, one must be attentive and slow down all mental and physical activity. To achieve this mental state, one may use breathing by following its length (breathe in-breathe out). Remember, *Tao Yin Han* requires breathing in through the nose and breathing out through the mouth while producing the sounds.

Relaxation: To relax while performing the postures and movements one must focus the attention on the relaxing sensation in the muscles and joints. An excellent way of experiencing immediate relaxation is through consciously smiling and keeping your attention on the smile.

Energy blueprint: This is a fundamental aspect of any *Qigong* practice. The idea of keeping the energy within the body needs to be understood. According to *Taoists* traditions, *Qi* flows throughout the body via the meridians and these energy paths crisscross the entire body and are also present on the surface of the skin, this is why certain body parts must be moved or blocked to allow the energy to flow freely or to remain within.
For instance, the "tongue", except when sound is produced, its tip must remain touching the hard palate throughout the practice. The palate offers a large area where to place the tip of the tongue, from behind the front teeth to near the throat; it all depends on personal comfort.
Armpits and groin (*Kua*) must remain open to let energy flow freely. When the pelvis is tilted in the perineal muscles and sphincter are lightly tighten up. The same happens when tilting in the chin; since the glottis sphincter is lightly tighten up as well. These two gates or locks are crucial for guiding the *Qi* within the orbits.
Another element is a *mudra. Mudras* are circuits formed with the hands and fingers. These *mudras* allow the energy to concentrate on specific meridians, and in more advanced practices they communicate certain energy qualities or characteristics. Also, a *mudra* communicates spiritual truths.

Once the student or practitioner begins his/her *Qigong* movements, the "eyes" should follow the hands wherever they go. Although it is possible to perform the movements having the eyes closed, even though, the eyes must follow the movement of the hands. There is an intimate connection between the mind (attentiveness) and the eyes as windows of the mind, while the hands are moved by energy. Remember, "energy follows thought". This connection prevents distractions and enhances the attentiveness.

Another possibility arises if you rather practice with your eyes closed and direct the eyes toward the tip of the nose, or to the point in between your eyebrows.

Since the *Kung Luohan* seeks to absorb and balance the *Yang* energy-polarity, throughout the practice we will always start our movements to or with the left (*Yang*) side, thus, moving first to the left side, placing our left hand inside the right hand when adopting the *Jieyin mudra*, etc., and finishing on the right (*Yin*) side.

Now, the following is a crucial aspect of how inner energy works, please pay attention to this matter. "Thought is faster than light", and we already know that "energy follows thought" instantly so, even if you are not thinking about the transmission of your *Qi* through your meridians, this inner energy is moving through them naturally and instantly and, it does not take time for it to flow and reach whatever energy path or energy center it goes to.

So, if you are performing an exercise, the *Qi* moving already through your meridian system will redirect its path through the selected orbit according to the *Li Zhang*, form or exercise and, it will flow through it without any effort, distraction or deviation, unless the energy path is somewhere blocked or saturated, which in that case, the *Qi* will seek to detour. This is why *Tui Na* is a helpful tool for removing all sorts of energy blockages and healing meridians.

Distractions: This is one of the most difficult aspects to eradicate. Distractions arise mainly from within and very little from the environment. The mind is quick to respond through reaction to even the slightest external provocation. Distractions are part of the environment internally and externally, thus, students and practitioners must enforce their will and avoid getting attracted to and distracted by thoughts-emotions arising from external factors.

Awareness is the only way the student and practitioner may avoid distractions. Awareness comes from a higher state of consciousness that allows the individual to presently observe whatever happens around and within him without been affected, thus, avoiding reactions (extra movements) that break the flow of *Qi*.

Awareness is the gate for entering into a realm of mental stillness. This process of stilling the mind may be a slow one but it is a transcendental mental state. If you feel discouraged, remember that stilling the mind is the gate into a brighter realm where new ways of perceiving and understanding everything lay.

Readiness: When you had reached a calm mental state you will understand that the use of intense muscular contractions, excessive stretching, or aggressive movements are counterproductive; thus, relax and breath naturally, slow and deep. Move slowly and ground yourself like a tree; flow free like a stream of water. Be soft like grass blades and do not oppose, do not crash, do not find yourself in conflict with anything or anyone. Free your mind of mundane worries, and harvest calm and internal peace.

Give yourself the chance of not thinking. Allow yourself to listen to and feel your body and enjoy the pleasure of being in tune with your physical Self during the movements. This is the way to remain in the present, in "the eternal here-and-now", yet fully conscious of your environment through your senses. Feel an alert, calm and detached awareness. This is *Sung* (meditation), which denotes relaxation, mental awareness, sensitivity, conscience, calm, loosening and tranquility of mind. Stay centered and in contact with reality!

Keep in mind that each posture and movement presents a specific way of doing it and that, for mastering it you must practice with proper care, no matter how simple it may look. Remember that moving parts like joints have a natural way of moving and a natural curvature so do not overstretch them or attempt to move them against their normal bend. Always keep all joints flexed naturally, never fixed or locked. Your spinal cord and its protective cover, the backbone must be straight as much as possible and we achieve that posture by tilting in both, pelvis and chin.

Never exaggerate your physical abilities and be mindful of your body and mind. Do not imitate others and become aware of your own strengths and weaknesses. Do not worry about your level of practice or ability; at the end, your knowledge of the forms is all that matters.

You must personally experiment through your approach to *Qigong* "treasures", which will develop your own understanding of body-mind cultivation. Without daily practice and without effort, the true knowledge will never occur.

Natural and reverse breathing; This is just a reminder about this sensitive element. In our *Qigong* practice we breathe naturally, deeply and slowly, however, we follow two main breathing methods employed by most *Qigong* and *Yoga* Masters, adepts and students. Although, it is true that most humans seem to have forgotten how to breathe,

these methods are fundamental for achieving a calm, quiet, and still or meditative mental state.
In earlier paragraphs I have presented a thorough explanation of this method called natural, which is the natural way all humans breathe when they are born. However, the reverse breathing method or *Taoist* breath is a bit more complex but with a little practice and attention can be mastered easily. Inhaling through the nose we bring the fresh incoming air to the top of the lungs by sucking in the abdomen and then we keep filling them to the bottom. This method does not inflate the abdomen but slightly the chest. When exhaling, the lungs deflate thoroughly by applying some pressure to the ribcage and popping out the abdomen until lungs are totally empty and free from toxins.
Although, it may sound difficult to practice, *Qigong Li Zhang* or exercises promote by themselves the two breathing methods without much concern about them.

Preliminary and final movements: There may be countless ways of beginning and ending your *Kung Luohan* routine. Generally speaking, our routine is preceded by opening or preliminary moves called *Qi Shi* to activate or organize the *Xian Tian Qi* or internal and external *Qi* field, and end with finishing moves called *Shou Shi* to guide *Qi* back to the lower *Dan Tian.*
You may perform some martial arts movements or adopting some particular *mudras*, perhaps you rather stretching a bit or bowing showing respect. It is up to you and the same happens with the end of your practice. Usually, when you practice with a group, the *Sifu* has his own way of starting and ending the practice.
Feel free to do whatever you feel proper. However, whatever you do must help you to relax your mind and

body, and to activate the *Xian Tian Qi* for practicing the movements and guiding the *Qi* to *Tan Tien.*

The following are the most common *Qi Shi* moves for achieving physical and mental calm and *Shou Shi for* concentrating the external and internal *Xian Tian Qi* within your body:

(1) "*Wu Ji*", Pillar or Column stance. It is fundamental and essential to do it to achieve mental, emotional and physical calm. It is upon this calm that internal *Qi* is activated and external *Qi* is absorbed.

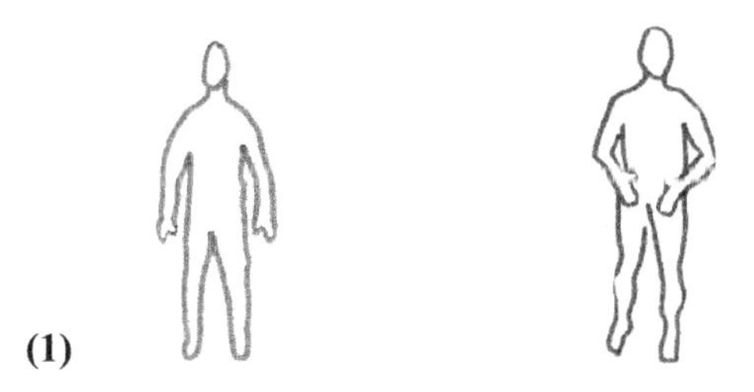

(1)

(2) "*Daikou*" or ***Dakku.*** It is a way of concentrating in the abdominal (*Tan Tien*) area the energy recently activated through *Wu Ji*, and which is moving within and outside the body through the energy mechanisms and the internal energy centers and meridians.
While at *Wu Ji* stance place both hands overlapped (right hand upon left hand) over *Tan Tien*, apply a slight pressure over the navel and take a few seconds to feel it. You may also feel on your left palm the pelvic bone just below the belly button.

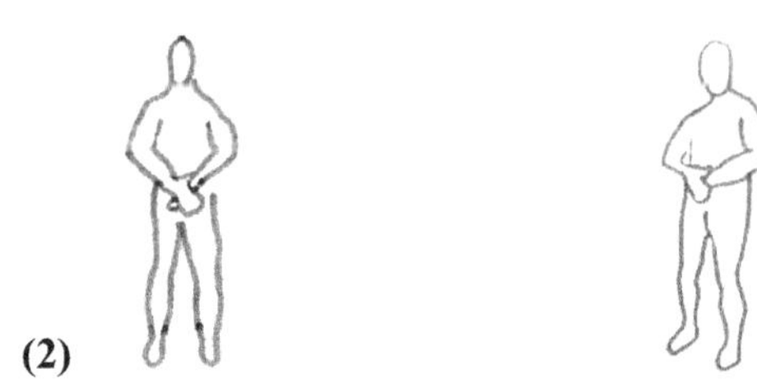

(2)

These two preliminary movements when practiced together are known as "Organizing the field & harvesting *Qi*": I always practice these two movements as *Qi Shi* prior to begin each section, and at the very end of the routine as *Shou Shi*. I strongly recommend including them in your daily practice. Both movements help to promote physical and mental readiness and tranquility.

(3) "Horse Stance". It is perhaps the most common posture of all martial arts. It is entered into it by moving the left leg-foot to the left (opening *Kua*), while the chin and pelvis are tilted in. The level of the stance will depend on the width of the base and the low of the center of gravity (pelvis-abdomen). This posture helps to maintain our back straight by pushing the pelvis forward, and slightly tightening the buttocks, perineum and pubis. From the energy standpoint, it helps to balance *Yin-Yang* polarities coming from earth and heaven when meeting and interacting within the body.

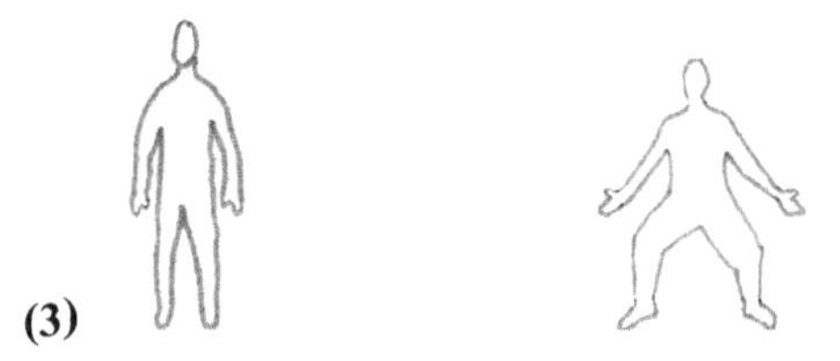

Final movements: Once you had finished your routine, practice *Shou Shi Daikou* by harvesting *Qi,* and finish it with at least three clockwise and three counterclockwise rotations of the overlapped hands. Both overlapped hands rotate around the abdomen, making a soft pressure upon it.

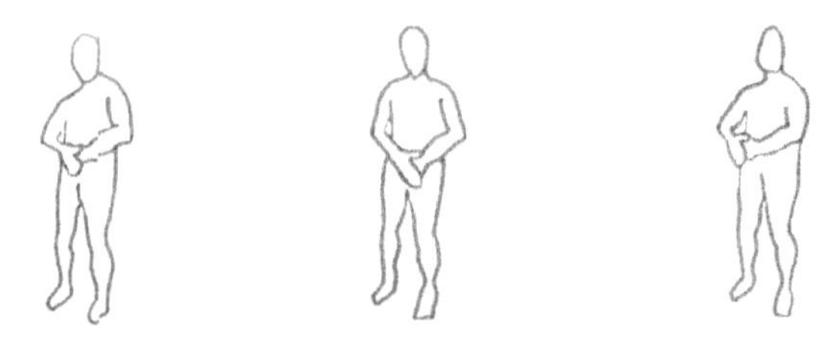

CHAPTER THREE

TAO YIN HAN
(KUNG LUOHAN, FIRST SECTION)

The preliminary movements will facilitate the activation of *Xian Tian Qi* (internal-external *Qi*) prior to start the *Tao Yin Han* routine.

The *Tao Yin Han* or first section of the *Kung Luohan* style is divided in seven exercises and each exercise is related to a specific orbit, meridian path, organ-gland, bodily system and sound. These movements also known as *Li Zhang* of the *Tao Yin Han* serve as a warm-up series of exercises before starting the *Ba Duan Jin,* second section or second phase of the entire *Qigong* practice.

You must practice all seven *Han* induction movements in order to relax your muscles, tendons and ligaments, vitalize the circulation of blood, lymph and *Qi,* while the six healing sounds will soothe, invigorate and heal all the five *Zhang* organs and the five *Fu* organs. This will effectively prepare the body for all forms of movements after the activation and distribution of *Xian Tian Qi*.

Tao Yin Han movements are suitable for any person regardless of age and, they can be practiced at any time. Also, they can help relieve work stress and uplift one's mental alertness. Just by practicing *Tao Yin Han* alone you can expel negative *Qi* from the body and thus, strengthen the body and the spirit.

Whether you practice the first and/or the second section, you should be able to feel the subtle *Qi* sensation on both palms (*Lao Kung*). Keep up with your practice faithfully so that your body can reach peak condition to receive the hidden wonders of the activation or *Xian Tian Qi*. When you reach this stage, you will mentally experience a state

that may last for days -- you then will receive the blessings of the Divine.
In this direct instruction method, there is an accumulative cultivation process. From now on, for the *Qi* cultivation process, you must practice all exercises daily. Practice in the morning and/or at night.
The series of exercises begin and end with the *Wu Ji - Daikou*, also seen as "organizing the field".

***1) Wu Ji** (Pillar or Column stance).

As mentioned earlier, this is both, the preliminary and final posture or stance we adopt every time we are about to begin or finishing our daily practice, therefore, it is a compound exercise or posture. It does not matter if it is the first or second sections or both; students and practitioners always begin with *Wu Ji* then, *Daikou.*
Also, this posture, although it is not necessary, sometimes is adopted in between exercises as a way of transition pose.
It is fundamental to practice it to achieve mental, emotional and physical calm, and it is upon this calm that *Xian Tian Qi* is activated or awakened from its dormant state.
This is a posture that represents "total void and calm" -- "the primordial condition" -- "emptiness and freedom from attachment, with no qualities".
It precedes all creative movement; it is the original expression (nothingness) before duality (*Yin-Yang,* both logically and temporarily).
The classic texts tell us that *Wu Ji* (the point in the center of a circumference) gives form to *Tai Ji (Yin-Yang).* In other words, emptiness transforms itself and it expands into the duality of the cycles (manifested expression of the Self), giving experience to the original creation.

***2) Daikou** (Harvesting *Qi*).

This is also a preliminary and ending movement and it is practiced as the final stage of the Pillar stance. It is also practiced with both, the first and second section or when practicing both sections consecutively.
This is a posture that concentrates or harvests the internal and external flow of *Qi* moving through the meridian system, and gathering or collecting in *Tan Tien* and through the external energy mechanism, which also connects with *Tan Tien*.

Performance:

- Adopt the regular horse stance (feet shoulder width apart), with toes slightly inclined inward and heels slightly outward. Relax all your joints lightly.

- Inhale while keeping a straight posture and lightly stretch the body and head buoyed up, as if an invisible thread is pulling you up. Chin and pelvis tilted in making the backbone straight. Exhale and relax all joints.

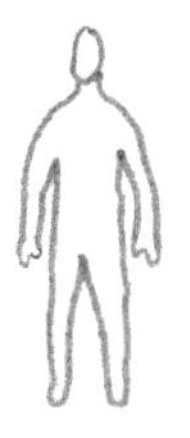 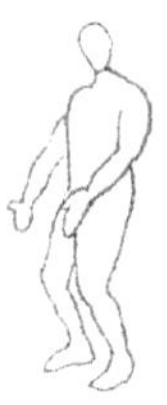

- Practice deep breathing in a soft, slow, deep and rhythmic way. Starting light and increase its depth; relax the body and mind with each breathing cycle. Relax your face but remain serene and content. Body moves up and down along the breath, inhaling-stretching up, and exhaling-shrinking down or bending the knees.

- Free your mind of thoughts, reduce internal chat and the flow of emotions, and focus in the present moment. Your sight should be relaxed and not focused on anything. Experience the sensation of *Qi* manifesting in *Lao Kung* and fingertips.

- Your lips must remain slightly touching without any pressure and your upper and lower teeth must remain slightly separated. Your tongue must be touching the hard palate.

- Your arms from shoulder to fingertips must remain relaxed alongside the hips, and relaxed with palms facing down-backwards. After few seconds of experiencing the *Xian Tian Qi* while at *Wu Ji,* and if you are about to begin your routine (either first or second section) then, you must adopt *Daikou* (overlapping right hand upon left hand and both upon the lower abdomen) to concentrate both, the internal and external energy mechanisms in the *Tan Tien* area.

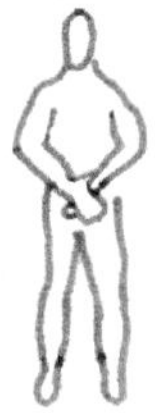

Note: Once your mind and heart become calm like still water then, you are approaching home.
Little by little your *Xian Tian Qi* will begin to be noticed as a vibration all over your body.
This posture permits the practitioner to connect to the universal *Qi* within and outside the body.

(1) TURTLE'S BREATHING (*Tuo Tian Bao Yue*).

Benefits: The movement improves the functioning of vital organs and glands within the abdominal cavity.
It works the lower back and waist muscles including the Psoas muscle as well as to oxygenates upper cervical vertebrae.

Relevant points: The movement allows the *Yin Qi* and *Wei Qi* to circulate the whole body. The *Yin Qi* stays inside the meridians, while the *Wei Qi* travels through and along the organs and reaching the skin and pores as a form of protection against the ill or cold wind and warm the body.
All joints are flexed during exhalation and stretched during inhalation.
The partial bending forward movement allows the *Qi* to stick to the *Yang* central meridian or the *Du Mai* channel, which is responsible for channeling the *Yang* polarity.
Both hands overlapped embrace (*Daikou*) the navel, pulling up the back, while eyes look down -- it should be performed gently and without haste.
There should not be any stiff point in the body so that the *Qi* can stick to the back (*Ming Men* acupoint aligned with the kidneys).
The "Heng" and "Huu" sounds are vocalized during the exhalation phase of the exercise.
This is the first of three exercises, which are performed having the heels together and tiptoes separated in a 45° angle.
This stance allows the moving *Qi* to remain within the body and flowing through the small orbit.

Performance:

(1) Starting at the end of previous form *Wu Ji,* and while still having the hands on *Daikou* then, bring both heels together and tiptoes separated 45° by pivoting the left foot to the left then, followed by the right foot to the right. *Daikou* will be maintained throughout the exercise.

(2) Inhale while legs, head are buoyed up and sight stretches up, and torso slightly stretches backward.

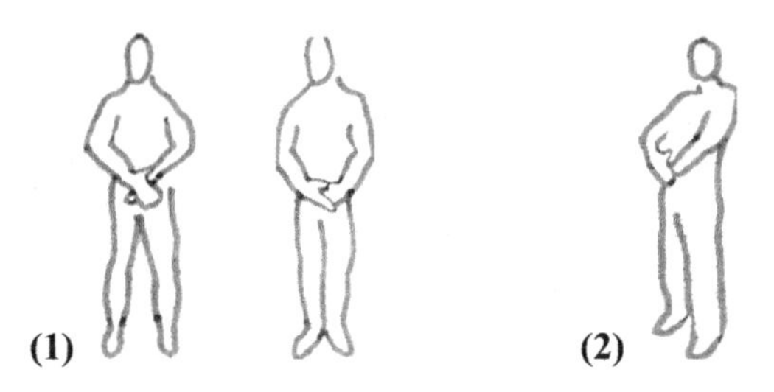

(3) Exhale while relaxing all joints and slightly bending the upper body frontally, and simultaneously producing the sound "HENG". Hands on *Daikou*, elbows move forward stretching shoulders, while hands press the lower abdomen sensing the pelvic bone.

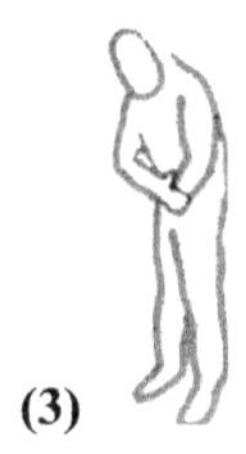

(4) Inhale while legs, torso, and head are buoyed up, sight stretches up, all while the torso slightly stretches backward.

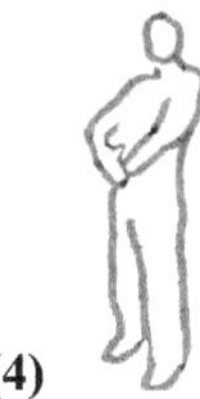

(5) Exhale while producing the sound "HUU" and start moving the left foot forward in a 15° angle; begin bending the torso toward the left foot. Hands on *Daikou* press over the lower abdomen and pelvic bone, while elbows move forward stretching.

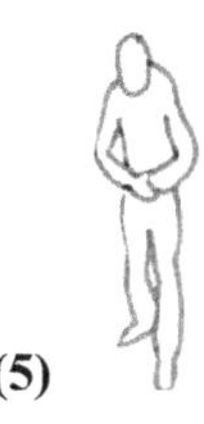

(5)

(6) Inhale while left foot moves back and legs and head are buoyed up, sight stretches up and torso stretches backward slightly.

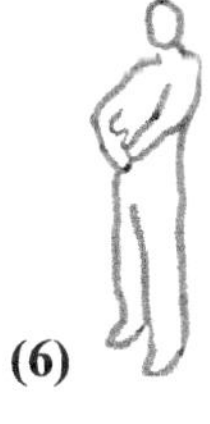

(6)

(7) Exhale while the upper body bends over frontally, and simultaneously producing the sound "HENG". Hands on *Daikou* apply pressure upon the pelvic bone; while elbows move forward stretching.

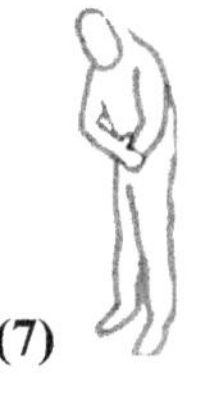

(7)

(8) Inhale while legs and head are buoyed up; sight stretches up and torso is stretched backward.

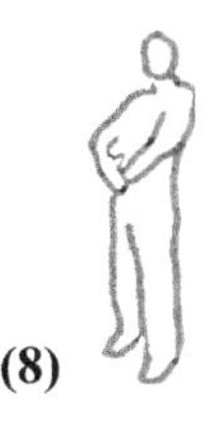

(8)

(9) Exhale while producing the sound "HUU" and start moving the right foot forward in a 15° angle; begin bending the torso toward the right foot. Hands on *Daikou* press over the lower abdomen and pelvic bone, while elbows move forward stretching.

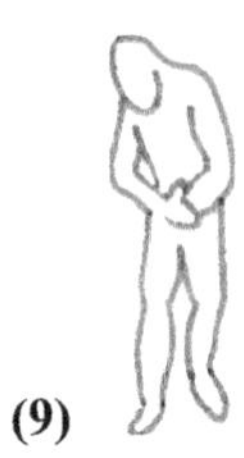

(9)

Note: Starting from number 2 and ending on 9, one cycle is completed. Repeat the cycle 3 times. After the third cycle is completed then, you are ready to move on to the next exercise.

Transition: After the last right step of the third cycle, just relax both hands resting on *Jieyin mudra* in front of the lower abdomen (left hand rests upon the right palm and thumbs tips touch each other). Heels remain together and tiptoes separated 45°.

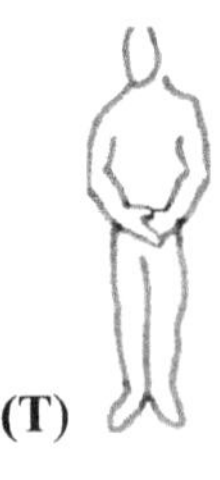

(T)

(2) HOLDING THE MOON (*Ying Feng Zou Bing*).

Benefits: Deep, slow and soft breathing helps to reduce blood pressure.
Stretching contributes to relax large muscle groups and increases blood circulation.
The posture helps to align the muscles of the back, the Psoas muscle and the backbone.
It is said that this exercise regulates and stimulates the functioning of all internal organs.

Relevant points: Start the movement with the sound "Heng" while your eyes look at the palms. When hands reach the highest point over the head immediately push up the whole body and begin the downward movement of the arms, followed by the sound "Ha". Throughout the exercise the eyes follow the hands.
The *Qi* naturally reaches the chest while producing the sound "Heng" and moves to the abdomen while producing the sound "Ha".
When both hands reach the highest point above the head, *Qi* has filled the chest and abdominal cavities and then, it flows freely through the *Sanjiao* meridian.
"Heng" and "Ha" sounds produce the kind of reverse breathing that comes naturally and which induces the *Qi* within the triple burner (head, chest, abdominal cavities and *Sanjiao* meridian). As result, the chest cavity will be soothing and the five *Zhang* organs are harmonized.
This exercise also raises the "*Shen*" (spirit) producing alertness.
The sounds "Heng" and "Ha" are vocalized during the exhalation phase of the exercise.
Joints are flexed during exhalation and stretched during inhalation.

Throughout the exercise the peripheral sight follows both hands, the head-face does not move at all.
This is the second of three exercises, which are performed having the heels together and tiptoes separated in a 45° angle. This stance allows the moving *Qi* to remain within the body.

Performance:

(1) Starting from previous ending or transition stance, the body's center of gravity sinks, pelvis and chin remain tilted in and hands adopt the *Jieyin mudra* (left hand resting inside the right palm, thumbs touching each other).

(2) Now, inhale deeply and slowly while the entire body stretches up.

(1) **(2)**

(3) Exhale softly producing the sound "HENG"; all joints are relaxed and simultaneously, both arms slowly sweep upward keeping both palms facing up and stopping once the fingertips of each hand almost touch each other above the head.
Do not move the head; however, the sight follows the hands throughout the ascending movement, immediately after and while still exhaling with the sound "HENG", heels, arms and backbone push up stretching the torso for about two seconds.

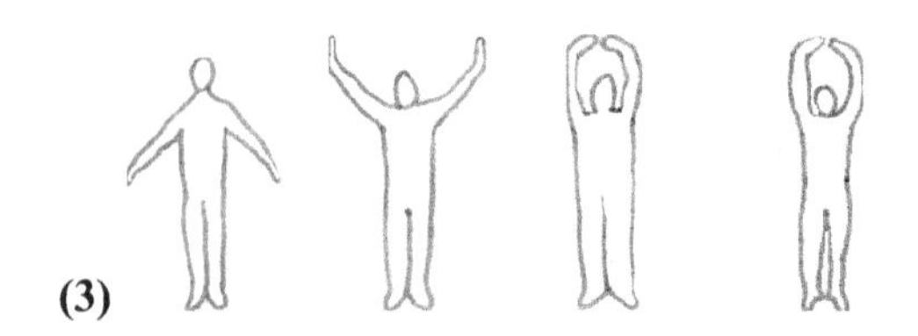
(3)

(4) Immediately after, the "HENG" sound changes to "HAA" while both arms begin a lateral slow descend. Keep pronouncing the sound "HA" until both hands reach the initial *Jieyin mudra*. Now your lungs are empty.

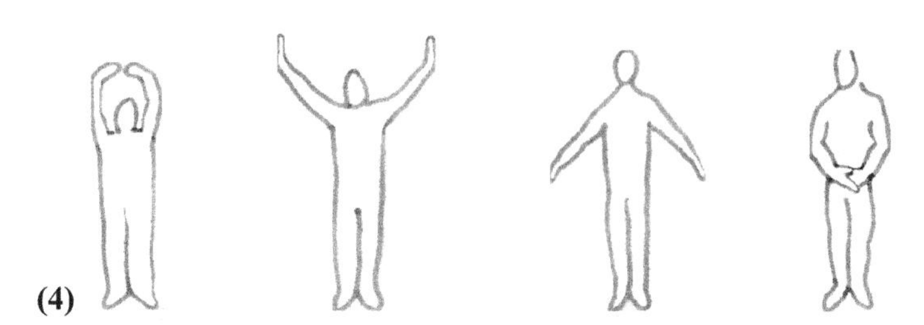
(4)

Note: Starting from 2 and ending on 4, one cycle is completed. Repeat 9 cycles before moving into the next exercise.

Transition: Remain relaxed with *Jieyin mudra* and the heels still remain together and tiptoes separated 45°.

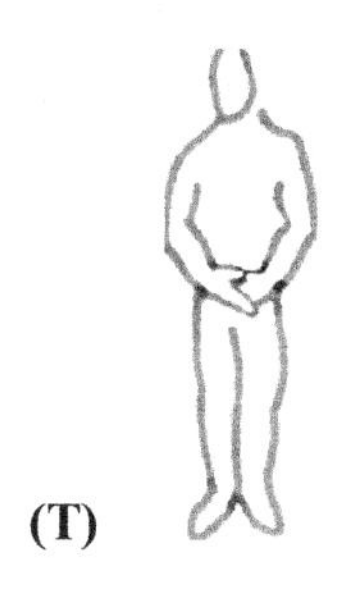
(T)

(3) DRAGON'S AWAKENING (*Fei Yen Hui Shou*).

Benefits: This posture works out the neck, shoulders and eyes muscles.
It balances brain functions, and movement coordination. Also it has positive effects on body's structural alignment; increases oxygenation of the blood and has a powerful effect upon the central nervous system, the circulatory system and the meridian system.
Lastly, this posture stimulates the kidneys' vital power, and it is excellent for reducing high blood pressure and it softens arteries.

Relevant points: The acupuncture point at the middle finger is the *Chong Liang* acupoint, which pertains to the gallbladder meridian. This meridian passes through the heart and when the heart and *Shen* (spirit) are mutually reacting the gallbladder benefits.
This movement is also called "the induction of the sight" and in it, *Qi* travels naturally through the middle finger meridian, which is connected to the heart and the gallbladder. Meantime by focusing the sight on the *Yi* (willpower) point at the tip of each middle finger the *Qi* is sensed in the five fingers.
With this exercise it is introduced the method of "recovering eyesight", which consists of staring at your middle fingers from one to three seconds, every time you stretch the shoulders and chest. Move the visual focus forward and backward between the middle finger and beyond by using *Yi Nian* or visualization.
If the shoulders experience some degree of ache after the third 180º head sweep, you can lower the arms adopting *Wu Ji* and resting for a few seconds before initiating the next cycle of three 180º horizontal sweeps.

The sound “Shui” or “Chuai” is vocalized during the exhalation phase of the exercise.
Joints are flexed during exhalation and stretched during inhalation. Every time the body stretches while inhaling, toes are also stretched and lifted opening *Yong Chuan* or ball of the foot acupoint, and the same happens with *Lao Kung* or palms.
This is the third and last of three exercises which are performed having the heels together and tiptoes separated in a 45° angle. This stance allows the moving *Qi* to remain within the body.

Performance:

(1) Starting from previous last or transitional stance, inhale and raise both arms frontally up to chest height, elbows out and palms facing the chest. Keep inhaling while both arms are turned outwards horizontally until both arms are stretched and fingers are lifted upwards.
While still inhaling, turn the face towards the left and focus your sight upon the left middle fingertip. Stretch back both shoulders and chest.

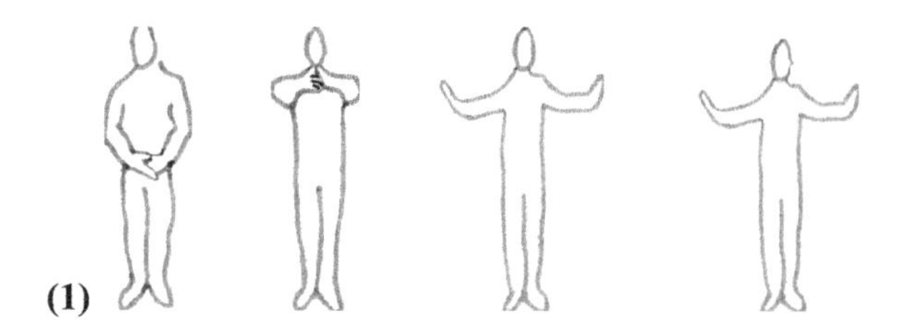
(1)

(2) Exhale while pronouncing the sound “SHUI” and begin turning the head toward the right side and relax the chest, shoulders and sight then, keep scanning the horizon until the face and sight reach the far right side then, focus the sight upon the right middle fingertip and stretch back both, shoulders and chest.

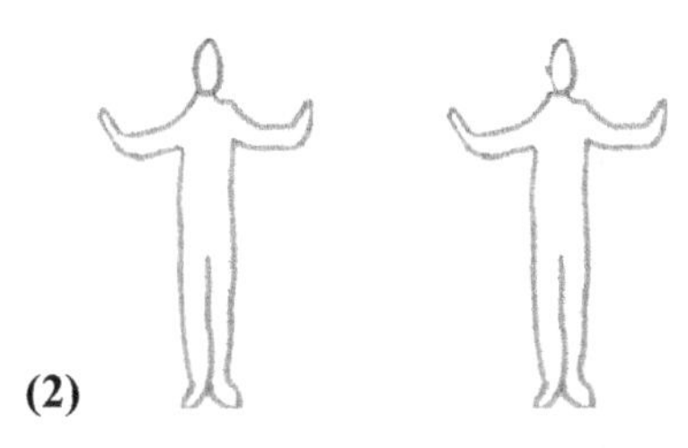

(2)

(3) Inhale and begin turning the face toward the left side and relax the shoulders, chest and sight then, keep scanning the horizon until the face and sight reach the left side then, focus the sight upon the left middle fingertip and stretch back both, shoulders and chest.

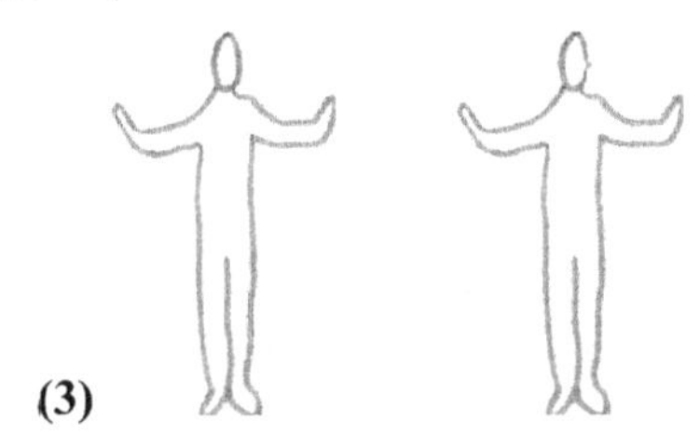

(3)

Note: Starting from 1 and ending on 3, one cycle is completed. Repeat three complete cycles before repeating it or moving into the next exercise.

Transition: After completing the third cycle's exhalation your arms are horizontal; begin inhaling and move them toward the center, aligned with the face; both palms face each other at the center. Begin exhaling while both arms descend toward the lower abdomen; the sight follows the palms, which are facing each other until reaching the lower abdomen. At this moment both heels move outwardly until feet become parallel shoulders width apart.

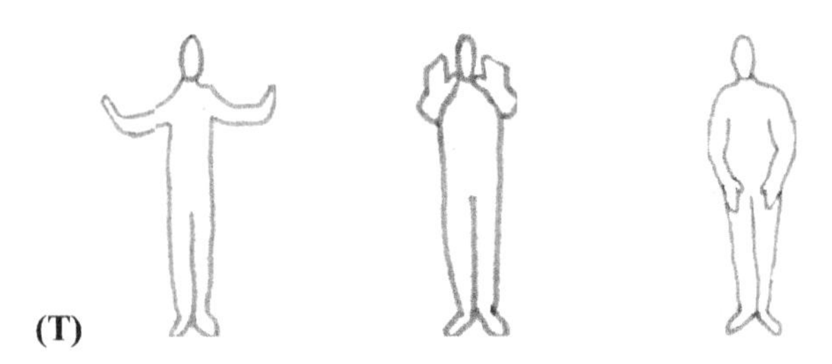

(T)

(4) CRANE'S FLIGHT (*Yao Bi Chao Tian*).

Benefits: Bones and tendons are strengthened, while the functions of internal organs become more efficient. Furthermore, nervous functions and upper joints are both improved and invigorated.

Relevant points: After the three previous exercises in which the stand demands for keeping the heels together and tiptoes separated, this is the first in which the feet are parallel with toes slightly inward. This way different orbits are now activated.

Sound "Ha" is produced with throat wide open merging the sound with the chest, which reverberates.

At the end of the third alternating left-right cycle, the transitional movement takes place. While inhaling raise both arms parallel above the head, which is buoyed up and palms face each other, then, exhale and bend the elbows until both palms face each ear.

After a few seconds *Qi* from the chest and abdominal cavities flow downwards gently and into *Kua* (hip joints and groin), then down to the knees and feet.

The *Qi* at the ankles will induce the four meridians of the *Yang Qiao* and *Yang Wei* to flow upwards through the sides of the body, and up to the elbows until they reach the palms. Then the *Qi* reaching both *Lao Kung,* react and attract mutually. This takes fractions of a second. Then, both hands descend following the energy mechanism along the torso until reaching *Tan tien.*

The *Yin* and *Wei Qi* flow surround the whole body. The *Yin Qi* circulates through the meridians and improves the transportation of nutrients in the blood. While the *Wei Qi* travels amongst the internal organs, reaching the skin and hair.

This exercise dispels "negative or ill wind" and warm up the body.

Performance:

(1) Inhale while both arms rise frontally and parallel, with palms facing each other until reaching above the head, all along the ascending movement the sight follows both hands.
The head does not move at all.

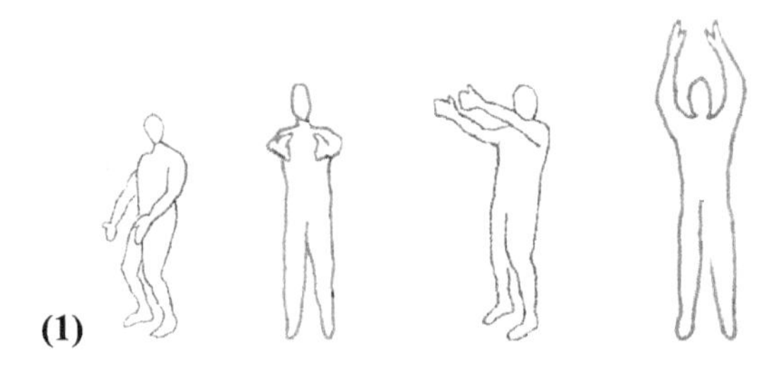

(2) Exhale while pronouncing the sound "HAAA", and simultaneously the face-neck turns to the left side stretching the neck and whipping out both arms, palms turn outward descending laterally.
The sight follows the left hand while descending rapidly until reaching initial position at *Tan Tien*.

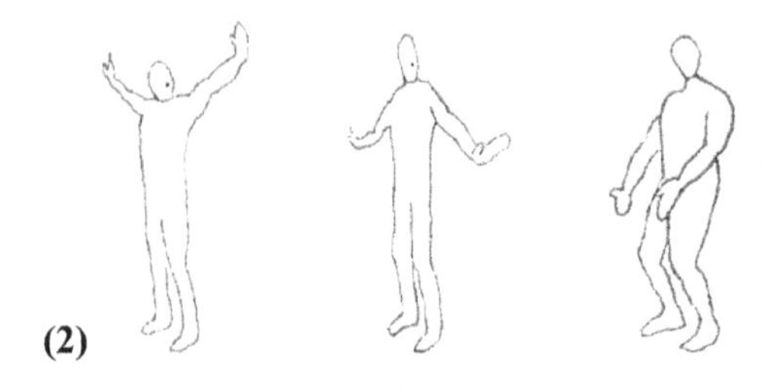

(3) Inhale while both arms rise frontally and parallel, with palms facing each other until reaching above the head, all along the ascending movement the sight follows both hands.
The head does not move at all.

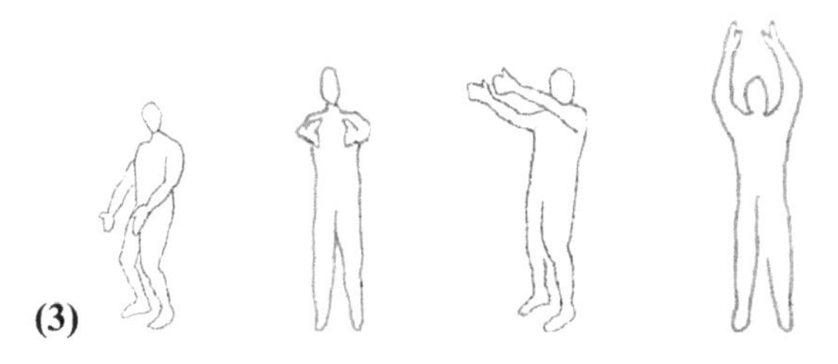

(3)

4) Exhale while pronouncing the sound "HAAA", the face-neck turns to the right side stretching the neck and simultaneously, whipping out both arms, palms turn outward descending laterally. Sight follows the right hand while descending rapidly until reaching initial at *Tan tien*.

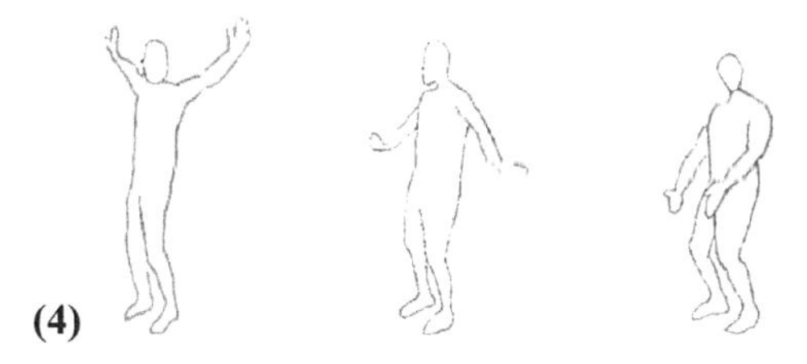

(4)

Note: Sarting from 1 and ending on 4, one cycle is completed. Repeat 3 alternate cycles before moving into the next exercise or repeat exercise.

Transition: Right after finishing the last third right whip, inhale while both arms rise frontally and simultaneously from *Tan tien* until reaching above the head, palms facing each other and eyes follow hands. Keep both hands above the head for few seconds sensing *Lao Kung.*
Then, start exhaling slowly while both hands slowly descend placing the palms in front of each ear, keeping them there for a few seconds while still exhaling and sensing the *Qi.* Then begin descending both palms toward the lower abdomen by starting facing the shoulders, the chest and follow the energy mechanism along the torso until reaching *Tan Tien.*

Toes are relaxed then, exhalation is completed and ready to move to the next exercise.

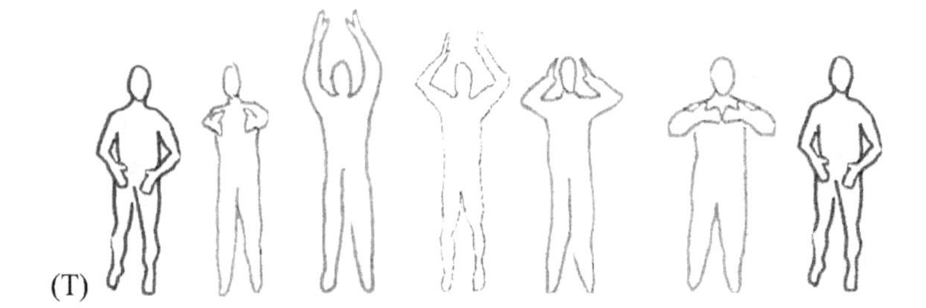

(5) CARRYING THE GREAT BASKET (*Yao Bo Ji*).

Benefits: Exercising the heart and lungs help absorb heat and prevents heartburn.
Lower horse stance posture strengthens legs, lower back and the Psoas muscle. Lumbar vertebrae are worked out.
Stretching also strengths pelvis, abdomen and upper back.
Spiral movements allow *Qi* to circulate freely allowing kidneys to receive and store large quantities of *Qi*. Tendons and ligaments are soothed.
This movement makes the pelvis joints agile and flexible.

Relevant points: This movement activates all acupoints of the body.
Blood, lymph and *Qi* flow smoothly and mood becomes cheerful.
The mental state and movements are constantly unified.
Relax and open the hip joints (*Kua*), knees and ankles are flexed to the lowest level by lowering the center of gravity.
Turn and pivot the hip joints, shifting the weight effectively to form twin circles -- like forming an "8" shape figure.
Maintain body's equilibrium by tilting in both, pelvis and chin. The head and trunk follow the turning direction of the hip joints. Body weight sways and rests on the hip joints. Elbows remain aligned with the sternum and palms facing up and slightly leaning toward each other, remain aligned with the knee.
Movements and technique must be constantly coordinated when swaying left and right.
Eyeballs do not move, remaining still and looking forward and level.
Through the spiraling movement of the spinal cord, *Qi* reaches the bottom of the feet attaching to the ground. This

will allow the *Qi* and bodily fluids to mutually merge and flow smoothly.

Performance:

(1) Starting from previous transitional *Wu Ji* stance and while still exhaling, adopt the lower horse stance by opening *Kua* to the left, aligning knees with feet at 45º angle, arms also open and hands remain just above knees without touching them, palms upward. Meantime, sight is fixed forward.

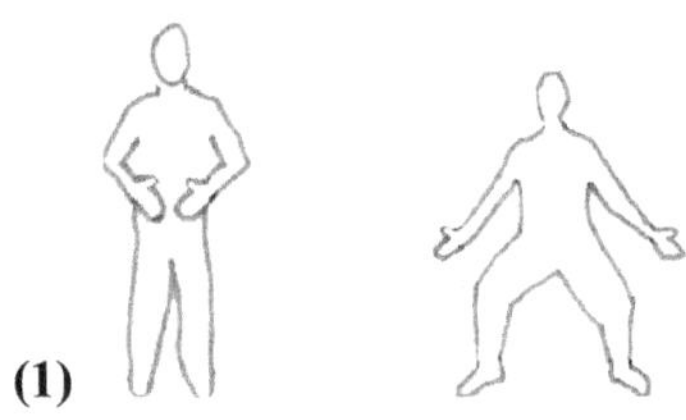
(1)

(2) Inhale while slowly rotate the torso and head towards the left. Shoulders and arms follow the torso toward the left, shifting body's weight towards the right leg-hip, slightly bending right leg while left leg extends partially; both arms and hands act as carrying a great basket. Rotate the backbone until reaching the far extreme of the movement.

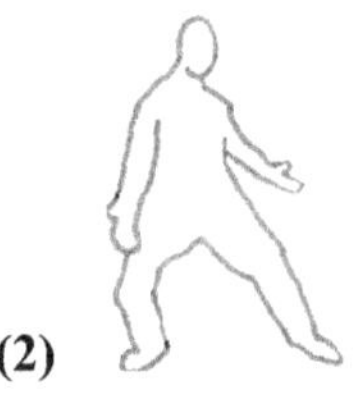
(2)

(3) Exhale while rotating to the right and pronouncing the sound "SHEE" until reaching the maximum turning extension. Shoulders and arms follow the torso toward the right, shifting body's weight towards right leg-hip, slightly bending left leg while right leg extends partially; both arms and hands act as carrying a great basket. Rotate the backbone until reaching the far extreme of the movement.

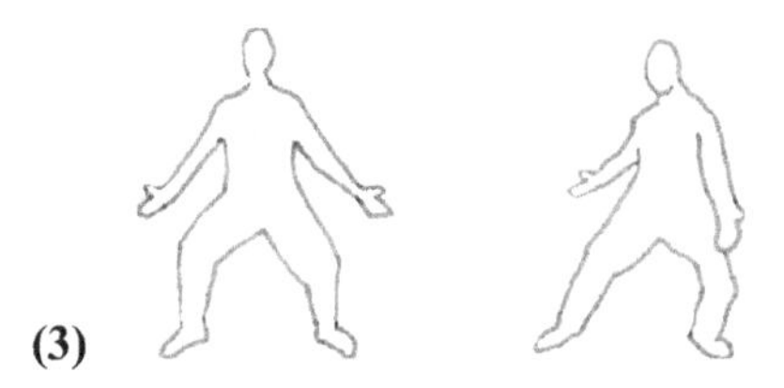

Note: Starting from 2 and ending on 3, one cycle is completed. Repeat 9 times or any multiple of 9 cycles before moving into the next exercise.

Transition: Once the last cycle is completed and while exhaling, close *Kua* from left to right, centering the body; arms should remain alongside the hip, hands adopt the "hollow fist" *mudra.*

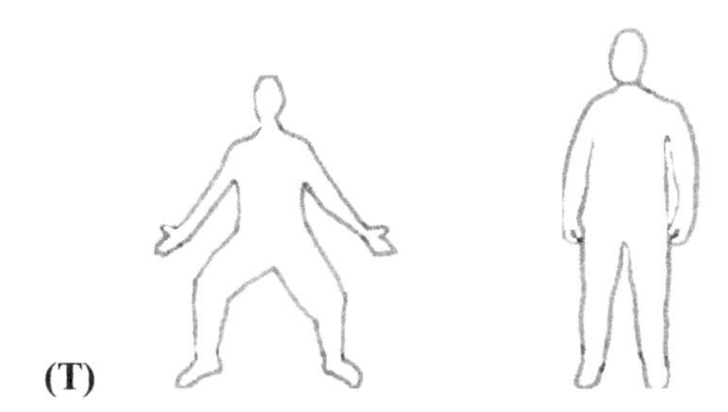

(6) PICKING GRASSES (*Ba He Shi*).

Benefits: The movement loosens and soothes ligaments and tendons, strengthens waist, legs, back and backbone. Also, it improves hepatic and cardiac functions and the brain becomes more alert.
This exercise energizes thighs, tendons and hipbones.
The chest and its internal organs expand in comfort. When the head tilts up the *Qi* stimulates the internal organs and causes them to feel relaxed and energized.

Relevant points: *Qi* moves to the chest and abdominal large cavities reaching the kidneys in a linked manner. This is beneficial to the energy level in the kidneys and intestinal area.
Also, this exercise allows the blood and *Qi* to flow smoothly, especially for people with a sedentary lifestyle.
Qi penetrates the hollow fists *mudra* and the body's external surface (skin). Hollow fists take place when folding the four fingers upon the palm and the thumbs press upon the fingernails of the already bent four fingers. This is referred to as the "empty fist", with the eye of both fists being the tunnel created by the curvature of the fingers. The eye of the fists must point forward, placing both fists alongside the hips.
All joints are slightly flexed while exhaling.
Head is buoyed up; arms, shoulders, back and sight lean backwards while inhaling.
When pronouncing the "Heng" sound, *Qi* reaches the lower abdomen and with the "Ha" sound, *Qi* reaches the kidneys. Pronounce the sound "Heng" from the throat and create resonance in the lower abdominal cavity then, pronounce the sound "Ha".

Performance:

(1) Starting from previous transitional stance inhale and begin stretching up. The head is buoyed up; arms, shoulders, back and sight lean up-backwards. Hands are already holding hollow fists.

(2) Exhale while bending over pronouncing the sound “HENG”, slightly tucking in the chin. The left hollow fist descends as much as possible trying to approach the toes of the left foot, or even touching the ground in front of the left foot.
Then the head gets raised, stretching the neck and gaze focuses between eyebrows, while right hollow fist remains beside the right knee without touching it.
Immediately and while still exhaling, switch the sound to “HAA” and begin the ascent, tilting the chin in and raising the torso to the original stretched standing and relaxed position, keeping both hollow fists alongside the hips.

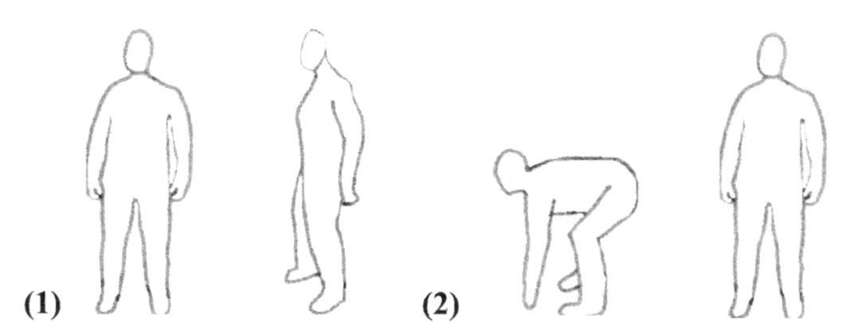

(3) Inhale, head is buoyed up, arms, shoulders, back and sight lean up-backwards. Hands are already holding hollow fists alongside the hips.

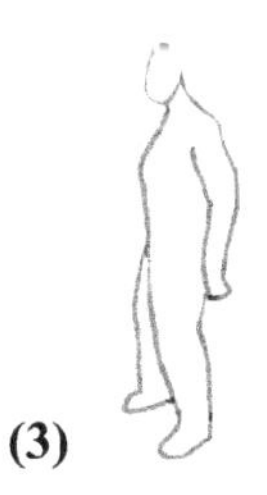

(4) Exhale while bending over producing the sound "HENG", slightly tucking in the chin. The right hollow fist descends as much as possible trying to approach the toes of the right foot, or even touching the ground in front of the right foot. Then the head gets raised, stretching the neck and gaze focuses between eyebrows, while left hollow fist stays beside the left knee without touching it. Immediately after and while still exhaling, switch the sound to "HAA" and begin the ascent, tilting the chin in and raising the torso to the original stretched standing and relaxed position, keeping both hollow fists alongside the hips.

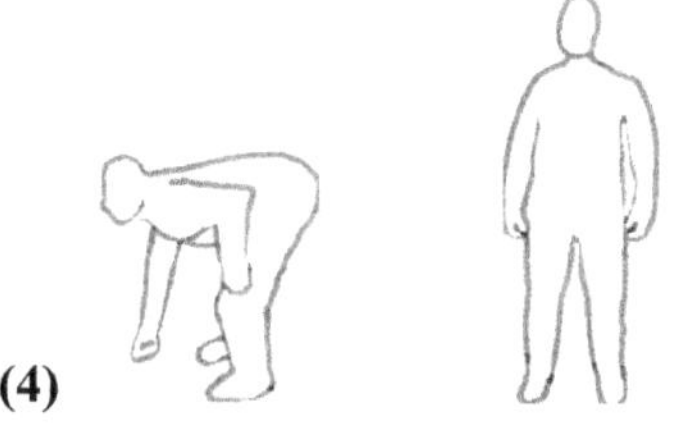
(4)

Note: Starting from 1 and ending on 4, one cycle is completed. Repeat this alternating exercise 9 cycles.

Transition: Once the ninth cycle is completed, remain calm, relaxed and with a straight stance for a few seconds sensing *Xian Tian Qi*, hands still in hollow fists hanging alongside the hips.
While sensing the *Qi* your body moves up and down following the rhythm of your breath.

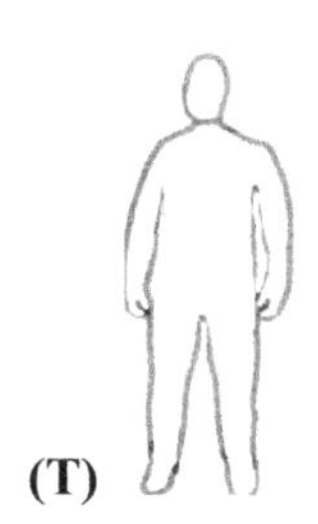
(T)

(7) BRIDGE BETWEEN EARTH & HEAVEN (*Fu Yao Shi*).

Benefits: These movements soothe the abdominal, chest and head cavities.
It strengthens the thighs, the lower and upper back and it stretches the torso.
Gravitational field transfers weight through bones, tissue, and muscle into the Earth. The Earth rebounds surging back up the legs, spinal cord and the brain, energizing, adjusting and animating posture, movement and exprcssion.
The posture and the movements become an uninterrupted exchange of conscious energy between the Earth, the Self and the Universe.

Relevant points: The sound "Huu" is linked to the tail end of the "Xuu" sound. With these two sounds *Qi* reaches the nerve endings of both hands and moves up to the back part of the brain. Seek to merge the two sounds with the back of the chest cavity.
Vibrations of the "Hoo" sound penetrate through the skin of the skull.
You will feel soothing at the chest, abdomen, and the rest of the body.

Performance:

(1) Starting from previous transitional last stance and while still holding hollow fists, inhale, the head is buoyed up and arms, shoulders, back and sight lean up-backwards.

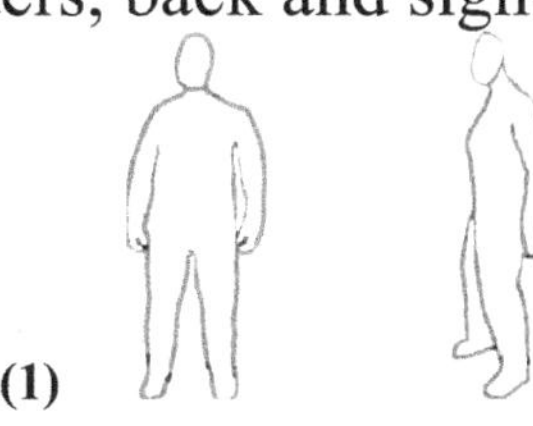

(2) Exhale and bend over, keeping the back as straight as possible; descend into a full squat and pronounce the "XUU" sound, while the eycs remain focused on the tip of the nose. Hollow fists should reach the ground alongside the ankles. At that lowest point, the head raises and gaze still remains focusing on the tip of the nose. Slightly, tuck the chin in and gently buoy up.

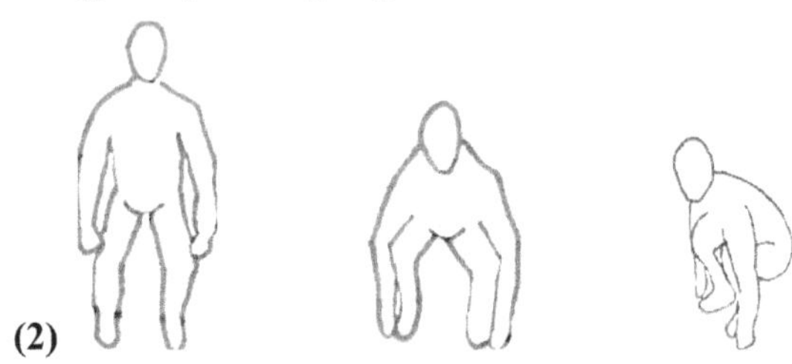

(3) Inhale slowly while rising from the full squat and straighten the torso and legs; the eyes remain focused at the tip of the nose. Once straighten up, hands are placed in front of *Tan Tien* with palms facing to it.

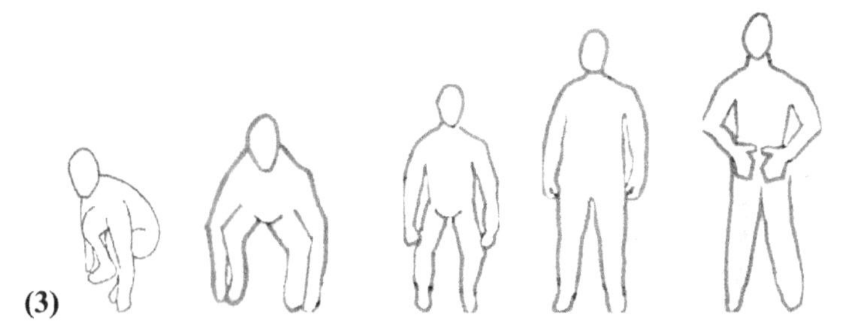

While still inhaling open *Kua* to the left side adopting the lower horse stance then, immediately rise the left arm until the palm faces the front of the left ear without touching it, fingers pointing upward and elbow remains outward; Simultaneously, move the right arm to the waist line, left hand remains leveled with the rib cage without touching it, palm facing the torso and fingers pointing downward and elbow remains outward.

Both hands are pointing in opposing directions (up and down) and the sight now moves to the point in between the eyebrows.

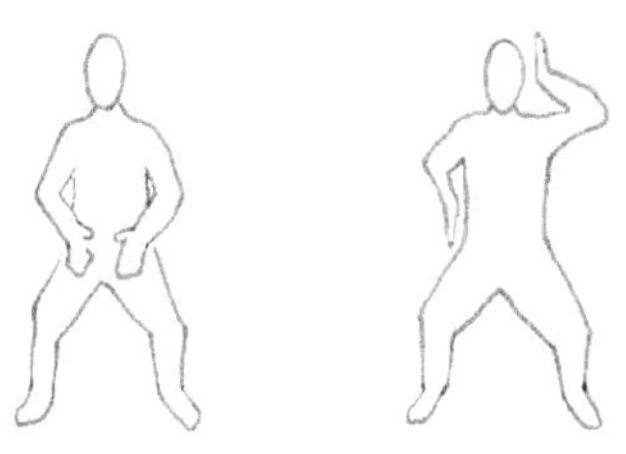

(4) Exhale while pronouncing the "HUU" sound, and stretch both arms in opposite directions. Sight remains locked in between eyebrows.

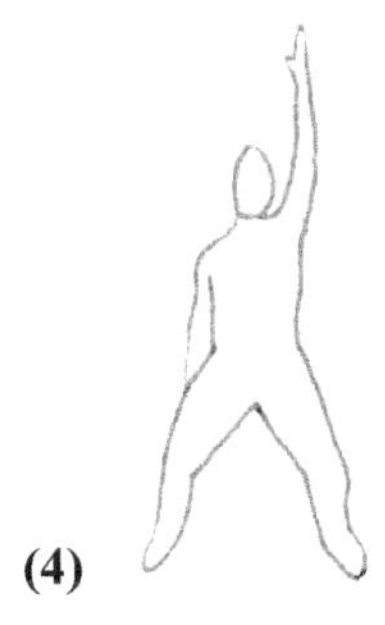

(5) Inhale while both arms return to *Tan Tien* with a fluid movement, place both palms in front of *Tan Tien* then, close *kua* to the right and move back to the initial standing stance, keeping both hands into hollow fists; head buoyed up, arms, shoulders, back and sight lean up-backwards.

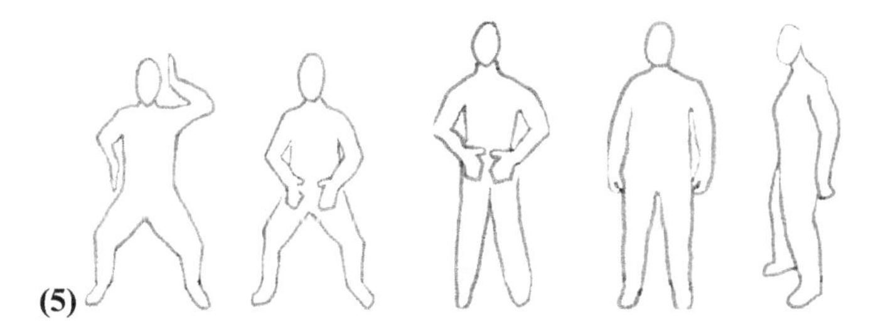

(6) Exhale while bending over keeping the back as straight as possible into a full squat and while pronouncing the "SHUU" sound. While the eyes remain focused on the tip of the nose. Hollow fists should reach the ground alongside the ankles. At that lower point, the head raises and gazc switch between eyebrows. Slightly tuck the chin in and gently buoy up.

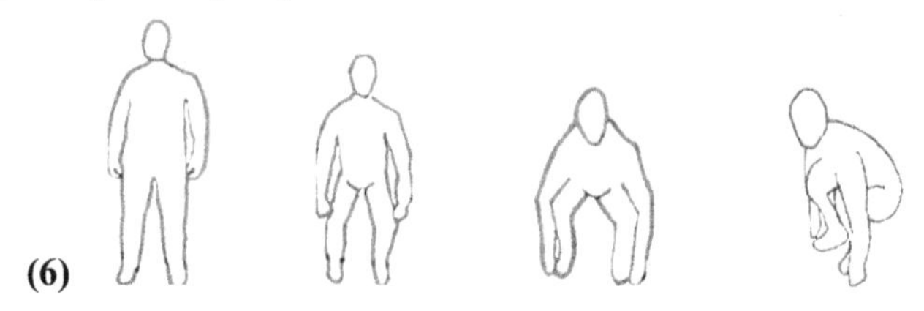

(7) Inhale while slowly rising from the squat and straighten up the torso, the eyes remain focused at the tip of the nose. Once straighten up place both hands facing *Tan Tien.*

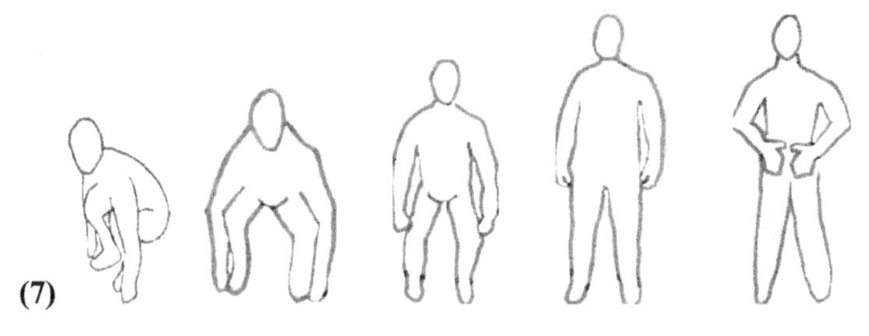

While still inhaling open *Kua* to the right side adopting the lower horse stance then, raise the right arm until the palm reaches in front of the right ear without touching it, fingers pointing upward and elbow is outward; Simultaneously, move the left arm to the waist line, leveled with the rib cage without touching it, palm facing the torso and fingers pointing downward and elbow outward.
Both hands point now in opposing directions, while sight moves to the point in between eyebrows.

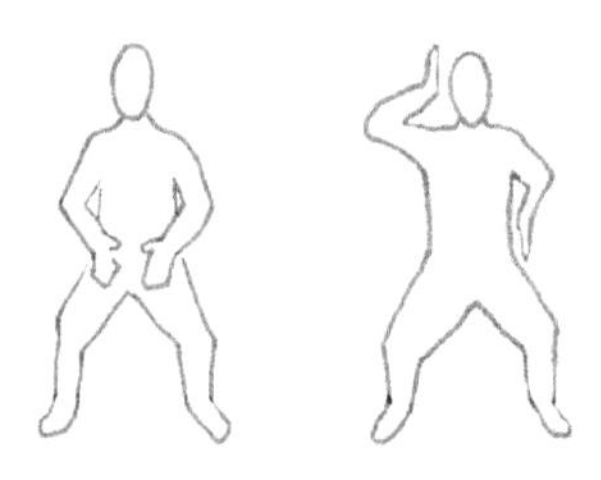

(8) Exhale while pronouncing the "HUU" sound, and stretching both arms in opposite directions.

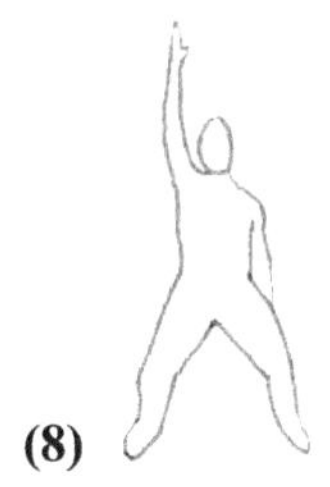
(8)

(9) Inhale while closing *kua* to the left and moving back to the initial standing stance, keep hands into hollow fists along the hip, head buoyed up, arms, shoulders, back and sight lean up-backwards.

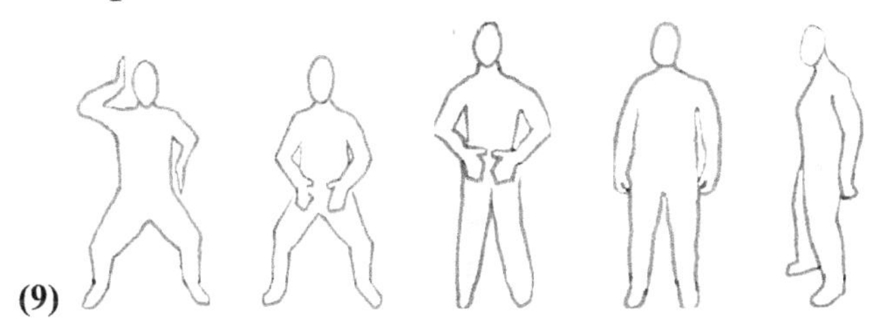
(9)

Note: Starting from 1 and ending on 9, one cycle is completed. Repeat 3 alternating cycles before moving into the next exercise.

Transition: Inhale while adopting the *Wu Ji* stance and relax sensing the *Xian Tian Qi.*

This is the end of the first section *Tao Yin Han.*

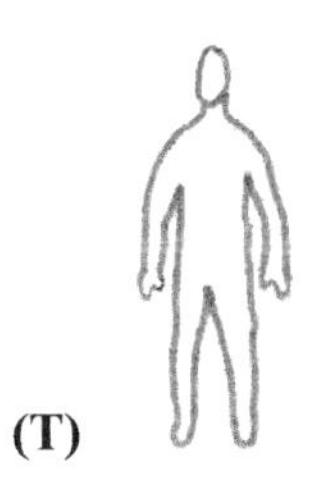
(T)

KUNG LUOHAN FINAL NOTES:

Congratulations for having completed the first section of the *Kung Luohan* style. The internal and external *Qi* are now active and the healing sounds have done their part, now you can go on with your everyday life. Your body and mind will begin experiencing the benefits of the activation of *Xian Tian Qi*.

Remember to keep practicing everyday and if possible, learn the second section, which will supplement and enhance your *Qigong* routine and health benefits.

In case that you still do not know the second section then, right after you finish your *Tao Yin Han* routine you may practice the supplementary movements in case you feel any excess of energy that can be translated as dizziness, or shortness of breath. If nothing of this sort is experienced then, you may practice sitting meditation focusing on the inner energy just activated through your *Tao Yin Han* practice, or practice the *Tui Na* acumassage if known.

It is highly recommended to learn and continue practicing the second and third sections called *Ba Duan Jin* and *Tui Na*. The *Ba Duan Jin* style of the *Kung Luohan* system is presented in the second volume and the *Tui Na* in the third volume of the series.

Yu Bei Shi or *Tai Ji Chi* exercise should be practiced either way, at the end of the first section or at the beginning of the second section in case each section is practiced separately. Nonetheless, if both sections are practiced one after the other then, *Yu Bei Shi* must be practiced in between both sections.

Yu Bei Shi is the first exercise of the second section known as *Ba Duan Jin*.

SUPPLEMENTARY MOVEMENTS

Although it is not necessary to practice these movements, it is my opinion that, in case you experience some kind of discomfort, like dizziness, tiredness, overheat or shivering after finishing your *Kung Luohan* routine then, practice the following supplementary movements. Experiencing any of the above mentioned uncomfortable conditions does not mean anything wrong, it is a natural body response so, do not worry since they will fade away very soon.

When one experiences any of these conditions or symptoms it is due to the excess of energy moving within the body, caused by the practice of *Tao Yin Han* and/or *Ba Duan Jin*. Generally speaking, these unpleasant conditions disappear almost immediately and once the body gets used to the stronger flow of energy that runs through the now widened meridians, wellbeing will be experienced.

In case you want to add these movements to your daily practice, do it right after finishing your full or partial *Kung Luohan* routine. If you know and practice *Tui Na* then, do these supplementary movements just before practicing *Tui Na*.

The supplementary movements serve to balance the energy moving within the body, also to eliminate any exceeding energy polarity. An added value of these movements is that they help to relax stressed joints, ligaments, tendons and softening meridians and lymphatic nodes right after practicing the *Kung Luohan.* You can practice them all one after the other, or picking any of them.

It is fundamental to understand that for obtaining the full benefits of *Kung Luohan*, it is necessary to practice your routine daily. It does not matter if it is only the *Tao Yin Han* section and/or the other sections and the supplementary movements. If you do not practice what

you learn, nothing is going to happen, nothing will improve and you would have wasted your resources.
Something else that you must seriously take into consideration is that, once *Xian Tian Qi* gets activated, each posture, each movement and each technique possess a unique response that you must discover and experience through committed practice. However, you must be sincere and honest to yourself and be mindful, remaining tranquil when you are nurturing your *Qi*.
Your perseverance will be prized once *Xian Tian Qi* gets activated, it will protect your body and mind keeping away all sorts of afflictions.

A *Taoist* principle says:

"If your heart is pure, your *Tan Kung* will also be pure. *Tan Kung* will reflect in your face the freshness and tranquility of your pure heart".

(A) Lifting knees: This is also known as "marching on the same spot". Lifting the left leg and then the right leg counts as one cycle. The movement is slow and with cadence. This movement adjusts and aligns the backbone, making it supple and promoting *Qi* flow in the central meridians.

Adopt *Wu Ji*.

First, raise the left knee to abdomen level, keeping the heel above the rest of the foot, which is parallel to the backbone, or keeping a 90° angle with the floor. Afterwards, lift the toes surpassing the heel and slowly descend the foot. The heel leads down the foot until reaching the ground.

Once the foot has landed and is parallel with the other foot, relax both knees.

Second, raise the right knee to abdomen level, keeping the heel above the rest of the foot, which is parallel to the backbone, or keeping a 90° angle with the floor. Lift the toes surpassing the heel and slowly descend the foot. The heel leads down the foot until reaching the ground.

Once the foot has landed and is parallel with the other foot, relax both knees.

Repeat the movement from 9 to 36 alternate steps. You can add arms swing movement, which needs to be synchronized with the legs, alternating the left leg with the right arm and, the right leg with the left arm. This exercise resembles a full march or military marching.

(B) Sidekick: Lifting the left ankle and then, the right ankle count as one cycle. The movement is slow and with cadence. Keep your arms alongside the torso.

Adopt *Wu Ji*.

First, lift the left knee just below the groin and turn the leg outwardly to the left side, just like preparing for side kicking. Hold the leg horizontal.
Turn your face to the left and see your left ankle above your left shoulder.
Lower the left leg and land the foot parallel to the right foot.

Second, lift the right knee just below the groin and turn the leg outwardly to the right side, just like preparing for side kicking. Hold the leg horizontally.
Turn your face to the right and see your right ankle above your right shoulder.
Lower the right leg and land the foot parallel to the left foot.

Repeat the movement from 9 to 18 times (alternating lefts and rights). This movement improves eyes mobility, soothes the legs tendons and improves legs flexibility. It also relieves waist pain.

C) Robot walk or the Pendulum: Lifting the left foot and the right foot count as one cycle. The movement is a slow alternating tilting, slowly advancing forwardly and then backwardly with cadence.

Adopt *Wu Ji*.

First, slightly lift the left foot forward and barely open *Kua* to the left. Place the left ball-of-the-foot on the ground and shift the weight of the body upon the right leg.

Slightly lift the right foot forward and place the ball-of-the-foot on the ground, shift the weight of the body upon the left leg.

Your will be moving slightly ahead and after the eighth cycle, stop and move backward repeating the steps.

Second, slightly lift the left foot backward and barely open *Kua* to the left. Place the left ball-of-the-foot on the ground and shift the weight of the body upon the right leg.

Slightly lift the right ball-of-the-foot backward and place it on the ground, shift the weight of the body upon the left leg.

Repeat the movement from 9 to 18 times (alternating lefts and rights). This exercise balances any exceeding energy. Once finished the last short step, relax for 60 seconds on *Wu Ji* while sensing the internal *Qi*.

FINAL NOTES

In order to obtain information regarding any of the topics covered by the books of this series, and/or if you want to contact *Kham Rel*, feel free to make contact through any of the following means:

Email: **zenbythelake@gmail.com**

Facebook: www.facebook.com/ZenByTheLake

Website: **www.zenbythelake.wixsite.com/qigong**

IS QIGONG AN ART?

Some people disagree with the idea that *Qigong* can be seen as an art. However, I think it is possible to understand *Qigong* as an Art expression. When a person practices *Qigong* with devotion, caring and honesty among other qualities, that person becomes an artist, simply because these are the same values that a consummated painter, dancer, writer or sculptor among others shows in his/her artwork.

The artist expresses himself through his own knowledge, his own internal and external resources and through creativity he produces something that communicates concrete or subjective ideas, feelings, concepts and abstractions. The artist also builds a vision of life, which is unique according to the way of expressing it. Furthermore, although the artist can use methods, mechanisms, tools and even theories to substantiate his artwork, the final result always transcends beyond the sum of all these factors.

Without any doubt, the artist is influenced by culture and he tends to reflect upon moral, philosophical, religious, economic, environmental, social, historical and political values or principles in the production of his artwork. Due to this positive thinking, the artwork results in a piece of art, which has intrinsic value and not necessarily economic value. Furthermore, if we add to the fact that Art can be understood as a synonymous of capacity, skills, talent and experience, we can see that all these elements also apply to the conscious practice of *Qigong*.

This way, when the artist has reached a certain degree of mastership in the use of those resources employed in his art field, along with the employment of those elements before mentioned, adding commitment and delivery, the final result is an expression of beauty and a fine piece of art.

When an individual practices *Qigong* his performance inherently includes devotion, caring, honesty, creativity, concrete concentration, abstraction, method, tools, cultural influence, capacity, skill, talent, commitment, delivery and experience, all conducive to mastership, which can be translated as Enlightenment due to the transformation or transmutation of his/her Self.

Khamrel.

Made in the USA
Middletown, DE
30 December 2022